Maria Fernes

THE FAMILY FOOT CARE BOOK

FOOT
CARE
BOOK
FOOT
CARE
BOOK
FOOT
CARE
BOOK
FOOT
CARE
BOOK
FOOT
CARE
BOOK

THE FAMILY FOOT CARE BOOK

Myles J. Schneider, D.P.M. & Mark D. Sussman, D.P.M.

ACROPOLIS BOOKS LTD.
WASHINGTON, D.C.

Dedications:

For Frankie and Sammy.

—Myles J. Schneider, D.P.M.

For Jenny.

—Mark D. Sussman, D.P.M.

ACROPOLIS BOOKS, LTD.
Colortone Building, 2400 17th St., N.W.
Washington, D.C. 20009

Printed in the United States of America by
COLORTONE PRESS
Creative Graphics, Inc.
Washington, D.C. 20009

Acknowledgments:
We want to thank the following individuals for their great energy and patience; Melody Sarecky, whose instructive drawings appear throughout the book and Monica Reid Spence, who cheerfully typed the manuscript (over and over). Finally, we would like to thank Alphons J. Hackl, president, publisher and editor of Acropolis Books, Ltd., for his belief in this project.

Drawings: Melody Sarecky

PRINTED IN THE UNITED STATES

Contents

Chapter 1

Introduction

A Note from the Authors

Dear Friends:

As podiatrists, we have always been interested in helping people who have problems with their feet to take better care of *themselves*, as easily and inexpensively as possible. The purpose of our book is not to provide theories or explanations of how the feet work, but to provide practical techniques for relieving pain and preventing it from recurring. We are delighted to have produced a guide which will not only show folks how to treat the problems they *can* treat safely and effectively, but also explains clearly and forcefully just what kinds of conditions require professional care.

At a first glance, a book on "self foot care" might appear to be against the best interests of the medical profession, as well as of the public. We have anticipated the objections that might be raised: that people who are not trained in medical care may do themselves more harm than good; that even if untrained individuals can safely care for themselves they might need more instruction than can be provided in a book; and—to be completely forthright—that books of this sort may compete with medical professionals for the consumer's health-care dollar!

We feel that all three objections can be addressed satisfactorily by simply pointing out that there are some 55 million Americans who need foot care services but have never visited a podiatrist's office. Since there are only some 8,000 podiatrists in the U.S., it is obvious that each one of us would be inundated with feet if all those who could benefit from our expertise decided to actively seek our help. More to the point, we would be so busy taping blisters and telling patients to replace those worn soles that we would be unable to give proper attention to the kinds of serious injuries or conditions that *must* have professional treatment.

What are the alternatives to a guide like this? With only a limited number of podiatrists available to treat millions of troubled feet, many of the people who walk (or hobble) on those feet will (1) turn to another kind of doctor who may not have the expertise and perspective necessary to provide proper treatment, (2) they will do nothing at all, simply letting their problems accumulate, or (3) they will attempt some sort of self-treatment. For those who would otherwise have no treatment at all, we think the value of a book which provides step-by-step guidance is quite obvious.

For those who might otherwise turn to professionals who are not specialists in foot care, there is more of a trade-off. On one hand, the patient may find a doctor who can provide better treatment than would be possible at home. On the other hand, he might walk into the office of a practitioner who would be more likely to rely on surgery or drugs than we would like to see.

But there is more than a question of "home-made" versus "professional" involved here. There is the broader question of how much each person in our society should assume responsibility for his own health. The traditional view is that such matters should always be left "up to the doctor," and that it is a mistake for any non-professional to meddle in matters that he would "not understand." But that view is changing rapidly. Our society's growing awareness of the value and all-pervasive nature of preventive medicine changes the picture completely around.

It is now apparent that *everyone* participates in his own health-care services *whether or not he or she intends to do so.* Every adult makes his own decisions regarding such vital questions as what nutrients will be taken into his body, what exercises his muscles will get from day to day, how much of that exercise will be aerobic, and so on. Relatively few people have any formal physiological or medical training on which to base such decisions, and few have the time or money to consult their doctors about such matters. Yet most survive, and it is partly because of the growing availability of basic health-care information (such as simple rules of good nutrition) that they do.

This book is not the product of any judgement on our part that medical information should be dispensed to the public. Rather, it is an outgrowth of our observation that people everywhere are *already in the business of taking care of themselves.* In the coming years, millions of Americans suffering from athlete's foot or blisters will "take their feet into their own hands" whether we podiatrists encourage them or not. Our job is not to encourage or to discourage them, but to help those who wish to do so by providing whatever specific information they may find useful. At the same time, we can help those who are enthusiastic about self-care to make careful distinctions between the kinds of problems they can cope with on their own, and those for which they need the services of a doctor. In each chapter, we have clearly indicated the conditions under which a doctor should be called.

As podiatrists, we have seen a tremendous growth of interest in preventive medicine and self-care during the past few years. Thousands of people we have met have often showed an ability to become quite expert at taking care of themselves. In fact, we owe many of the techniques and tips described in this book to them as much as to our own medical educations. We are highly confident of our readers' ability to take the information we have compiled here, and use it well. In doing so, we think they will not only save themselves the cost of medical bills they don't need (while freeing us to do the work we have to do); they will also have far more appreciation of the wonders and complexities of those remarkable feet they have fixed up than would have been the case if they had left the fixing to us.

Myles J. Schneider, D.P.M.
Mark D. Sussman, D.P.M.

Chapter 2

How to Use This Book

You don't have to know about medicine to be able to use this book. The whole idea is to help you get relief for your feet without the expense or inconvenience of going to a doctor.

Not all foot problems can be self-treated, however. To be sure that you are giving yourself the safest and most effective treatment possible, read all instructions carefully. Here is the sequence of steps to take:

1. Read the Guidelines to Treatment in this chapter. Take note of the kinds of conditions which require a doctor's attention, and *do not* attempt self-treatment on any of these. Notice that instructions are provided for various basic treatment techniques (such as icing and taping) which are prescribed in later chapters.

2. Also in this chapter, notice the "master list" of basic materials used in various treatments prescribed throughout the book. At the beginning of each chapter devoted to a specific condition to be treated, there is a list of "things you will need" for that condition. These "things" will be described in generic terms which may not always be familiar to you. For the names of familiar brands or inexpensive substitutes, turn to the master list in this chapter. For example, if the list of "things you will need" includes "soaking solution," the master list will show you that you can use either a solution of epsom salts or an inexpensive substitute—a solution of plain household detergent.

3. Once you have finished reading this chapter, look up the condition you wish to treat in the table of contents, and turn directly to the chapter indicated. Just in case you aren't sure what kind of condition you have, we have used descriptive names for our chapter titles. Each chapter starts off with a general description and sketch of the condition, which you should check carefully before proceeding any further.

4. Read through the entire chapter before beginning any treatment. If you do not understand the instructions, or if you are not certain what is wrong, or if you feel any reluctance to proceed with the treatment, see a podiatrist.

GUIDELINES TO TREATMENT

1. Contraindications (do not attempt self-treatment if you have any of the following):

A. Diabetes
B. Circulatory problems
C. Infection
D. Queasy stomach
E. Allergies or sensitivity to any of the recommended materials and medications
F. Poor eyesight
G. Unsteady hand

2. Precautions

A. Know your limitations. If you attempt a self-treatment and it does not improve the condition, see a podiatrist.

B. Follow directions for self-treatment as written. Do not overuse suggested medications or procedures.

C. Do not use any over-the-counter preparations other than those recommended in this book.

D. If during self-treatment you cause minor bleeding, apply a styptic as directed to control it. If bleeding is excessive, apply ice and compression to the area and see a podiatrist.

E. If you are instructed to use a heating pad for a specific problem, never use it in bed, and never at its highest setting.

F. Beware of frostbite: Don't use ice treatments for more than the recommended time periods.

3. Preparedness

A. Make sure any instruments you use are clean. Wash them in soap and water and rinse off with alcohol, Zephiran, Betadine, or some other recognized antiseptic.

B. Make sure all materials and suggested medications are clean and up to date. To sterilize any metal instrument, hold in a flame for a few seconds.

C. Scrub the entire foot thoroughly with warm soapy water and a terry wash cloth for at least one minute, and pat dry with a soft clean towel. For all of the self-treatments listed, this is sufficient preparation. However, if you care to, you may apply a mild antiseptic solution such as Sephiran chloride, Betadine, pHisoHex, or any other similar preparation.

D. To prepare for soaking, dissolve any of the following in one gallon of warm water: two domeboro tablets; two tablespoons of epsom salts; or two tablespoons of a mild household detergent.

Techniques You May Need

Many of the treatments described in this book involve the use of ice, taping, elevation, and other simple techniques. These techniques are explained here, rather than repeated in full for each of the many chapters where they are used. We recommend that you familiarize yourself with these techniques before beginning any of the individual treatments described in later chapters.

Ice

How to make it up . . . .

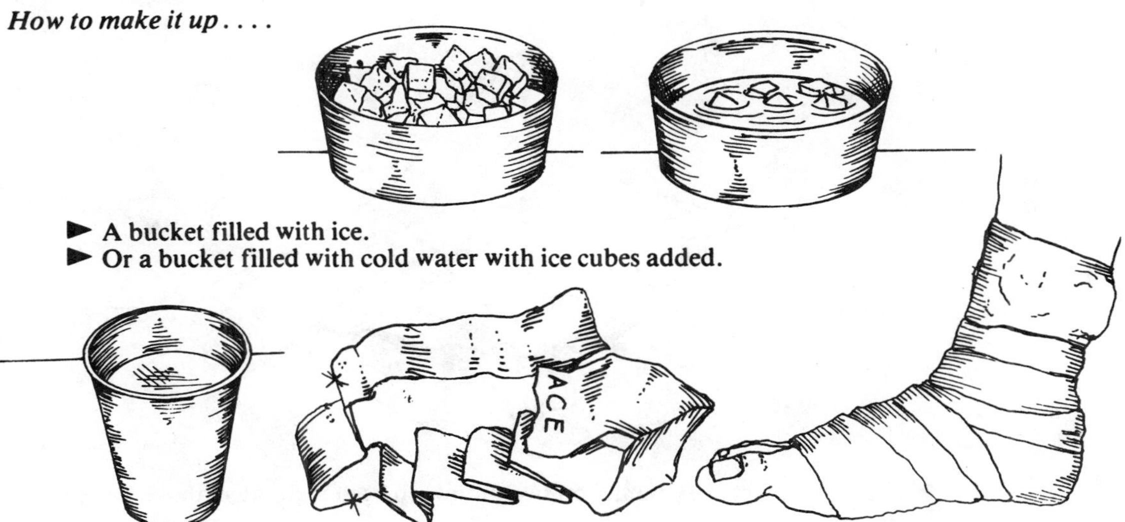

► A bucket filled with ice.
► Or a bucket filled with cold water with ice cubes added.

► Or fill a paper cup with water and freeze it into an easy-to-use ice applicator.
► Or soak an ace bandage in water and freeze it. Remove and put ice cubes over the painful area and wrap with the frozen ace bandage.
► Or if you have a home whirlpool, use cold water in it.
► Or soak a terry cloth hand towel in water, fold into a square and place in a plastic bag. Put it in the freezer until it hardens. The resulting ice pack can easily be used under an ace bandage.

How to use it . . .

► Apply 30 minutes on and 30 minutes off for the first three to four hours after an injury, or for a painful condition.
► For the remainder of the first 48 hours, apply the ice at least 30 minutes three times each day.
► After two days, proceed to ice *therapy.* Ice the area for six to twelve minutes or until numbness occurs, massaging it with the paper cup, ice towels or ice whirlpools, etc. Put the sore part through range-of-motion exercises (as recommended for specific conditions) until the pain returns. If the pain does return, replace the ice for six to twelve minutes. Then repeat the motion exercises. If no pain returns after five to ten minutes of active exercise, then re-do the ice for six to twelve minutes and stop. Ice therapy should be started no earlier than 24 hours and no later than 48 hours after the initial pain. The normal sequence of events is *ice,* exercise, *ice,* exercise, *ice.*

Elevation and Compression

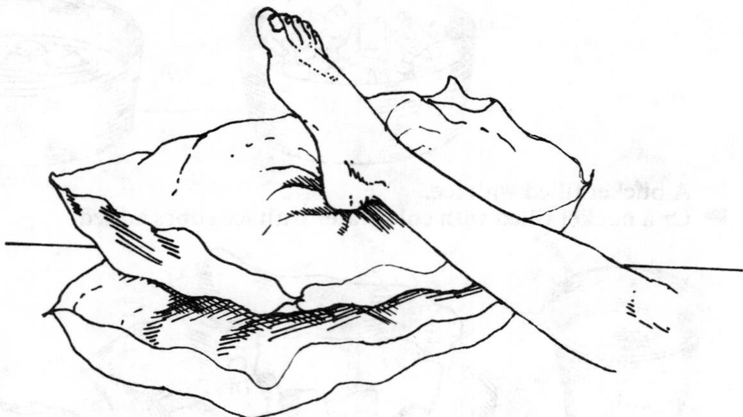

► Place the affected extremity on two pillows to keep it elevated above the level of the heart.

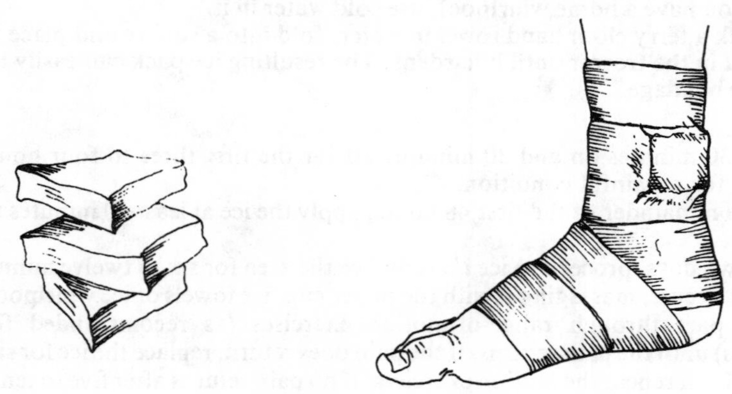

► Make a compression pad by cutting several thicknesses of foam rubber (approximately three inches by one half inch thick). Place over the affected area and wrap snugly with an ace bandage.
► Place ice directly over the compression pad.
► If the injured area (or the foot on that side) becomes numb or begins to tingle, loosen the compression bandage until the numb part is comfortable again.

Moist Heat Applications

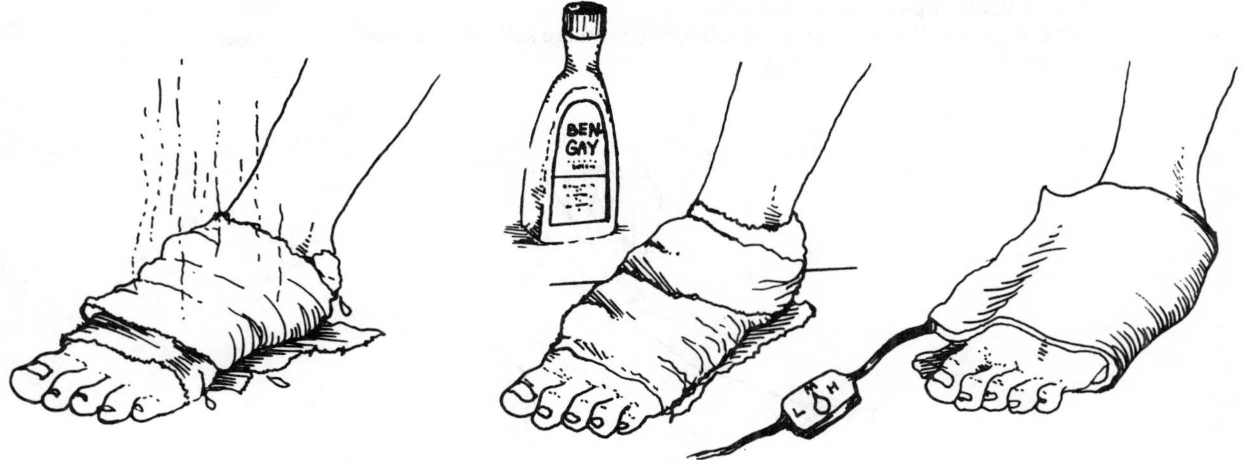

► Soak a towel in hot water and wrap it around the affected area for two to four minutes.
► Apply a heat-producing ointment like Ben-gay to the involved area, then soak a towel in hot water and wrap it around the area for two to four minutes.
► After the towel has cooled down, wrap a heating pad around the area for 15 to 20 minutes on medium heat.
► If you have a home whirlpool, use warm water, ninety to one hundred degrees Fahrenheit for fifteen to twenty minutes as an alternative.
► Use heat applications two to three times a day unless otherwise specified.

Aspirin

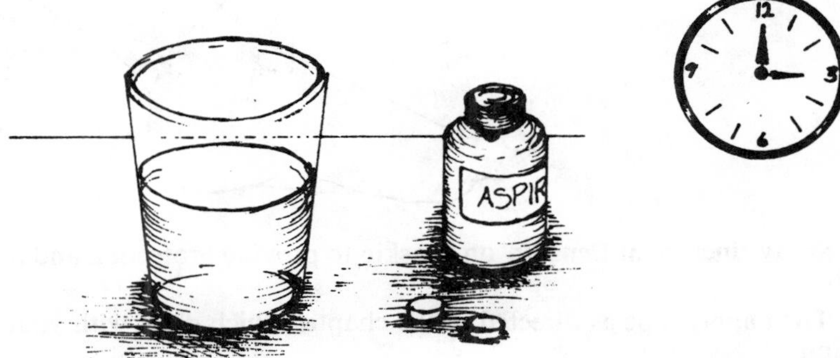

► To help eliminate inflammation and control pain, take two aspirin every four hours for two to three days and then two aspirin every six hours for up to a week thereafter, as needed.
► If you have an ulcer or an allergy to aspirin, or if you cannot take aspirin for any other reason, call your physician or podiatrist for an alternative method.
► Tylenol can be used to reduce the pain, but does not have the same anti-inflammatory properties as aspirin.

Taping

When using tape against the skin . . .

► Get yourself a good pair of scissors (bandage scissors are best).

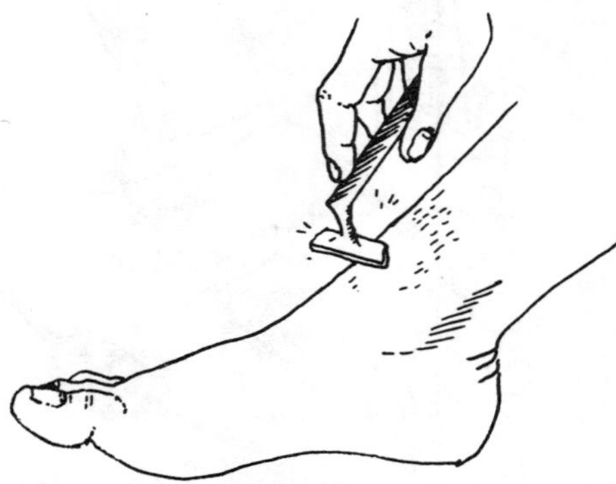

► Shave all hair from the area to be taped.

► Wash the area with soap and water before each application.

► Wipe the area thoroughly with alcohol on a cotton ball.

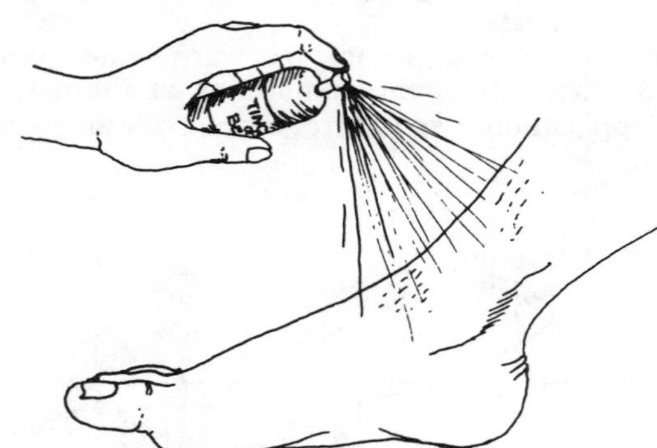

► Spray tincture of Benzoin on the skin to provide protection and help the tape adhere.

► Then apply tape as directed in the chapter which deals with your particular condition.

► After pads and tapings are in place, dust the taping liberally with powder to prevent sticking to socks and twisting of tape. As an alternative, rub a piece of paraffin over the tape.

► When you are using tape repeatedly, you can remove tape stains (the sticky greyish residue left when tape is removed) with hydrogen peroxide, nail polish remover, or acetone. Clean the nail polish remover or acetone off with rubbing alcohol, and wash with soap and water. This procedure will help to prevent skin irritation due to taping.

Exercise

► A *passive* exercise is one that is done without putting any weight on the part being exercised. It generally involves moving the foot or leg through a certain range of motion while sitting or lying down. An *active* exercise is one that is done while the part being exercised is actually bearing a full load as it normally would in walking or running.

Rest

► In the treatment of painful conditions, rest can be achieved in several different ways: It can mean pursuing all normal daily activities *except* those that put severe stress on the area (such as the stress of athletic training).

► It can mean *substituting* one activity for another (as in riding a bicycle or swimming instead of running).

► It can also mean putting *no* weight on the painful part (crutch walking). This type of rest would normally be prescribed by a doctor.

► In an extreme case, it can mean complete bedrest.

How to Remove Paddings and Tape

1. Soak in warm soap and water for five minutes to loosen.
2. Soak with baby oil.

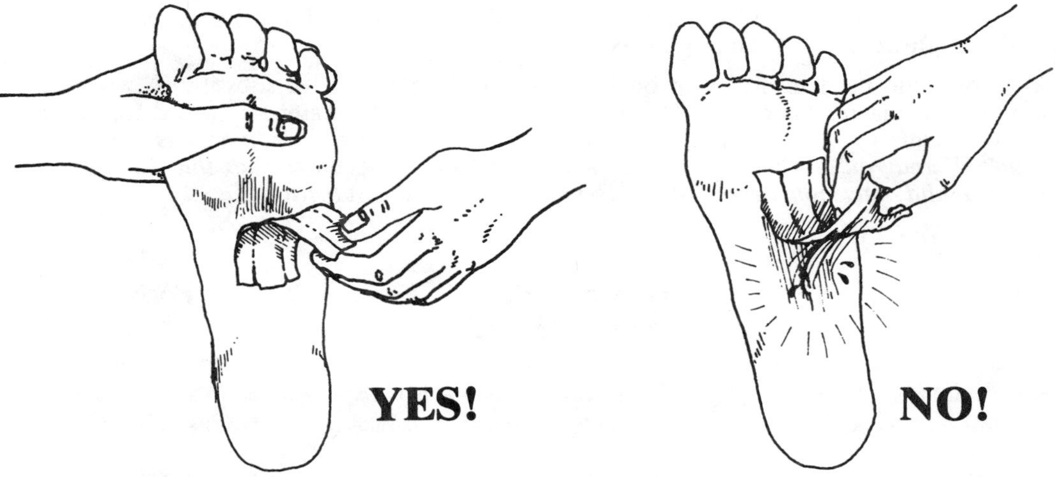

3. Always remove the tape slowly. When removing pads or tape on the bottom of the foot, *always remove in the direction of the heel*; otherwise you may tear the skin. With one hand, firmly grasp the skin just in front of the pad or tape; and with the other hand peel it slowly backward toward the heel.

► If you pull off pads or tape in the wrong direction and tear the skin, there will be bleeding and pain. If this occurs, do not be alarmed, but treat the wound as follows:

1. Do not cut skin away. Fold down in place.
2. Apply ice, compression, and elevation on two pillows for ten to fifteen minutes (see Elevation and Compression, above).
3. Once bleeding has stopped, apply an antiseptic cream. Cover with a 2"x 2" gauze pad and tape down. Remember, when removing *this* tape, pull it slowly *toward the heel* as suggested above!

Tape Allergy vs. Tape Reaction

Tape Allergy is a skin rash with itching, which will occur in susceptible individuals within a few hours after the first application of tape.

Tape Reaction is a skin rash with itching, burning, and blisters, which occurs only with repeated use of tape in certain individuals.

Treatment

1. Clean the affected area with soap and water. Pat dry with a terry cloth towel.
2. Apply Calamine or Caladryl lotion twice during the day and once just before bed.
3. Repeat step #2 until the skin reaction disappears.
4. If you have found that you are allergic to tape, remember to always use non-allergic tape in the future (and to tell any doctor who treats you that you have this allergy).

If the condition persists after three days of treatment, see a podiatrist. If severe itching, redness, warmth, blistering, and/or swelling occurs—or if pus formation occurs—see a podiatrist immediately.

MATERIALS LIST

At the beginning of each chapter we have listed the various materials and instruments needed for the treatment described in that chapter. Those materials are listed by generic names (rather than by familiar brand names) so that you can perform the treatment with maximum flexibility and at minimum cost.

For those who need information on brand names or inexpensive substitutes, we have provided the master Materials List below. This list covers the materials needed for all of the treatments described in the book. (*Example: if a particular chapter lists "soaking solution" and you don't have any epsom salts on hand, you can consult this list and see that any mild household detergent will serve as an acceptable substitute.)*

Item	*Generic or Inexpensive form*	*"Top-of-line" form*
ace bandage	store brand stretch bandage	**Ace bandage**
adhesive felt padding	homemade (felt backed with rubber cement)	**Scholl's**
adhesive foam padding	homemade (foam backed with rubber cement)	**Scholl's**
adhesive spray and skin protectant	tincture of benzoin	**Benzoin Spray**
adhesive tape	store brand adhesive tape	non-allergenic tape **(3M)** or "paper" tape **(Johnson & Johnson)** or porous adhesive tape **(Zonas)**
ankle brace	ace bandage or adhesive tape in figure "8" pattern (see chapter 37)	store-bought elastic ankle brace
antibiotic cream	a prescription item (may have around house)	**Neosporin Cream**
anti-fungal liquid	Tinactin liquid	**Tinactin liquid**
anti-perspirant	store brand	**Mitchum's**
antiseptic	Zephiran chloride, alcohol, or merthiolate	**Betadine**

antiseptic cream	first aid cream	brand name
aspirin		
baby oil	castor or mineral oil	**Baby Oil**
bandaid	gauze and adhesive tape or store brand plastic bandage strips	Johnson & Johnson **Bandaid**
bunion shield	make your own (see chapter 16)	**Scholl's**
calfskin or kidskin leather		
callous file	home-made callous file (see chapter 8)	callous file available in drug stores
corn pad, non-medicated	cut your own out of moleskin, felt or foam (see chapter 6)	**Dr. Scholl's**
cotton	hank or roll of cotton	cotton balls
cotton material 1" by 18"	rope or rubber band	
cotton swab	home-made cotton swab (blunted tooth-pick and cotton) or store brand	**Q-tips, Cotton Swabs**
desensitizing lotion	home-made paste (Baking soda and water or meat tenderizer and water) or **Calamine** lotion	**Caladryl lotion**
disinfectant spray	**Lysol**	**Desenex**
elastic adhesive bandage	non-elastic adhesive tape	**Elastoplast**
fabric for removal of dead skin	wash cloth or gauze pad	**Pumice Stone**
foot roller	soda bottle or rolling pin (do not subse-quently use for pie)	custom hardwood foot rollers **Footsie Roller**
2"x 2" gauze pads	store brand pads, available in discount and chain drugstores	**Johnson & Johnson**
heating pads	electric, cloth cover	electric, rubber backed
heat ointment	liniment, mustard plaster	**Ben Gay**
heel cup	rubber or plastic store bought	**M-F Heel Protector, Tuli's**
ice bag	paper cup of water, frozen, or terry hand towel folded, soaked in water, put in plastic bag and frozen	chemical "ice" bag
lamb's wool	wool shorn from your own lamb	store-bought lamb's wool
lipstick		
matches	matches	matches
material to inhibit odor	10% formaldehyde (as directed) solution	Johnson's "Odor-Eaters"
medicated foot powder	corn starch	**Tinactin or Aftate**
mildly abrasive tool	home-made abrasive tool (see chapter 6) or emery board	pumice stone
moleskin	**Dr. Scholl**	Dr. Scholl
nail brush	tooth brush	store bought nail brush
nail file	emery board, mildly abrasive tool (see chapter 6)	store bought nail file
nail forceps, straight back	cuticle forceps, available in drug store	straight-back nail forceps available from medical supply house
nitrogen-impregnated foam innersole	store brand innersole	**Scholl Sponge Foam** or **Spenco innersole**
non-adhesive felt		

occlusive wrap	sandwich wrap	**Saran Wrap**
paper	plain drawing paper	graph paper
paper clip		
petroleum jelly	store brand petroleum jelly	**VASELINE™ Petroleum Jelly**
pillow	2 pieces of material sewn and stuffed with feathers or foam	store bought pillow
pin, needle, or tweezers	sewing needle or straight pin	store bought tweezers
plastic wrap (air-tight dressing)	store brand	**Saran Wrap**
40% salicylic acid plaster	**aspirin tablets crushed and mixed with water to make paste—applied to wart and covered with adhesive tape**	**store bought**
scissors	**any old pair**	**sharp, bandage type**
slant board	**home-made slant board**	**Flex-Wedge**
soaking solution	Epsom salts (in solution as directed on box) or mild household detergent (in solution)	**Domeboro** or **Bluboro** tablets or powder, as directed
soap & water	home-made soap (made with lye and left over fat from cooking	anti-bacterial soap **(Dial)**
softening agent (vegetable oil)	vegetable oil	olive oil
soft polyurethane foam	kitchen sponge	
sponge rubber heelpad or raise	scrap of indoor outdoor carpet cut to size,	store-bought heel cushions
toothbrush	old toothbrush	new toothbrush
wet heat	towel soaked in hot water, rubber heating pad over wet towel	hydrocollator or whirlpool bath

Chapter 3

Ingrown Toenail

(Onychocryptosis)

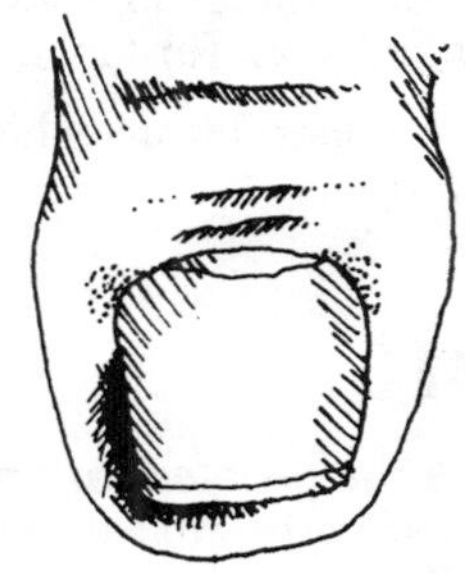
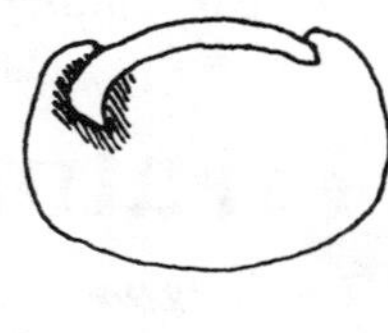

What is it?

An ingrown toenail occurs when the side of a toenail cuts through the surrounding skin. The area becomes very sensitive to pressure. Continued pressure may cause redness, swelling, and—eventually—infection. Nail pressure occurring over a long period of time may even lead to the formation of small painful corns in the nail groove.

Things you will need for this treatment

see chapter 2 "Materials List" for brand names and substitutes

soap & water
antiseptic
ice bag
nail forceps, straight-backed
2"x2" gauze pad
soaking solution
bandaid
antibiotic cream (if you have any)

Caution: *Do not proceed with this treatment until you have read the Guidelines to Treatment in Chapter 2*

Preparation for Treatment

► Make sure any instruments you use are clean. Wash them in soap and water and rinse off with alcohol or some other recognized antiseptic.

► Make sure all materials and suggested medications are clean and up-to-date.

► Put two tablespoons of mild household detergent into ½ gallon of warm water. Dip your foot in the water and soak for ten minutes.

► Read through all the instructions which follow, and make sure you understand them before beginning treatment.

Treatment

The *only* way to solve the problem of an ingrown toenail is to remove the ingrown part. Soaks and antibiotics are otherwise useless. An ice pack held against the toe (for no more than five minutes) will provide some numbness.

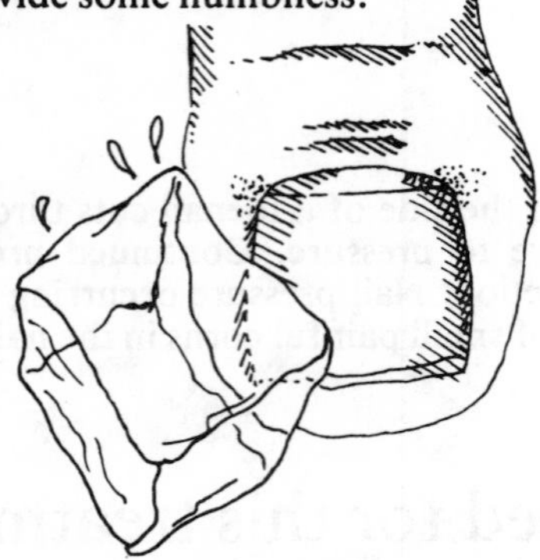

1. To remove the offending part of the toenail . . .

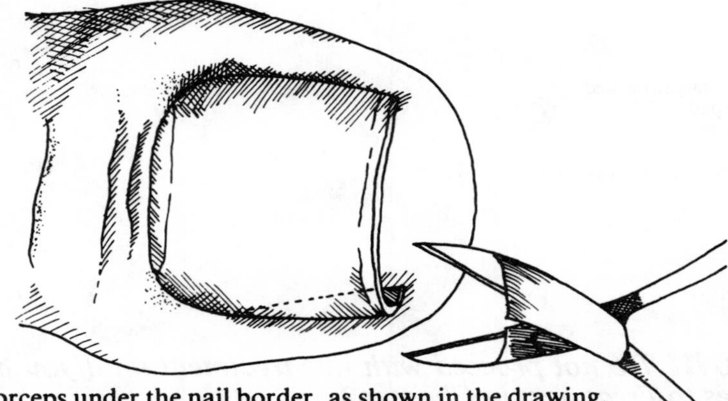

► Insert forceps under the nail border, as shown in the drawing.

► Clip out the ingrown toenail at a slight angle.

► Try not to cut flesh, by keeping the bottom of the clipper as close to the bottom of the nail plate as possible. *Hang in there!* It's normal for this to be a little uncomfortable.

► Try not to leave nail spicules (pointed fragments), as they will tend to start the ingrown process over again.

► Once the nail is cut, grasp the corner and gently pull it out.

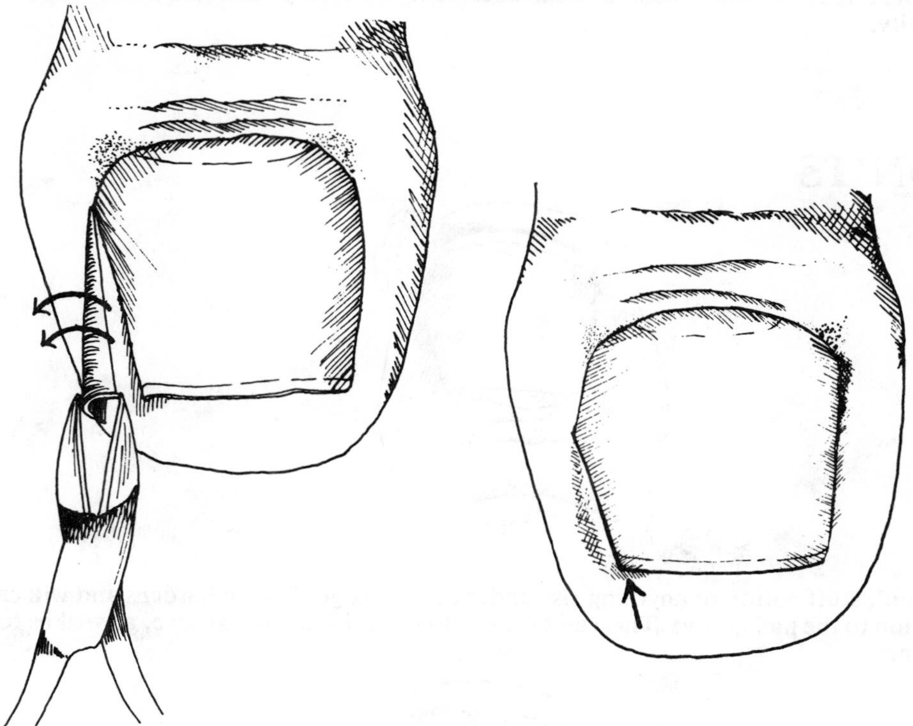

2. Wipe off the area gently with soap and water on a gauze pad.

   ► If there is bleeding, elevate the foot and apply an ice pack for ten minutes with light pressure. If bleeding is minor, you may use a styptic. If it is excessive, apply ice and pressure *and* see a podiatrist.

3. During the next few days...

   ► Until tenderness is gone, soak your toe for 20 minutes, twice a day, in one of the following:
   - Two domeboro tablets dissolved in one gallon of warm water
   or
   - Two tablespoons of epsom salts in one gallon of warm water
   or
   - Two tablespoons of a mild detergent such as Ivory Liquid, Tide, etc., in one gallon of warm water.

   After you soak, apply Merthiolate (which will act as a drying agent), a bandaid, and an antibiotic cream such as Neosporin (if you have any).

When to Call the Doctor

If pain is not reduced after one day, *or* if you have left a spicule (pointed fragment), *or* if you think you have an infection, see your podiatrist immediately. If the do-it-yourself treatment provides only temporary comfort and the problem soon returns, you can have the ingrown part of the toenail permanently removed by your podiatrist through a minor procedure that is done under a local anesthetic with very little pain and almost no disability.

DON'TS

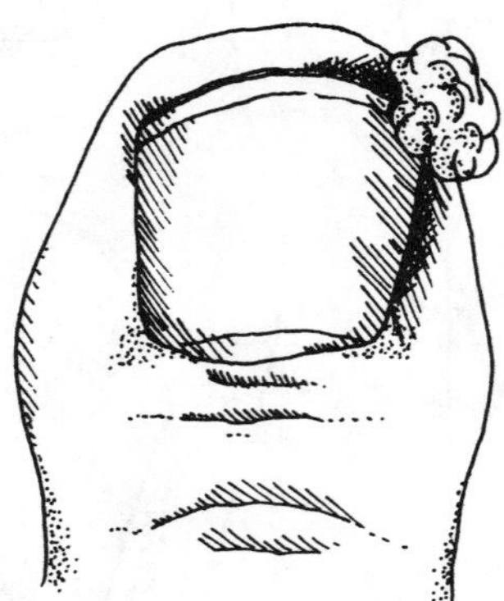

► Don't stuff cotton or anything else under the nail edge. Cotton hardens and will cause irritation to the nail groove This can give rise to corns in the nail groove, as well as to infection.

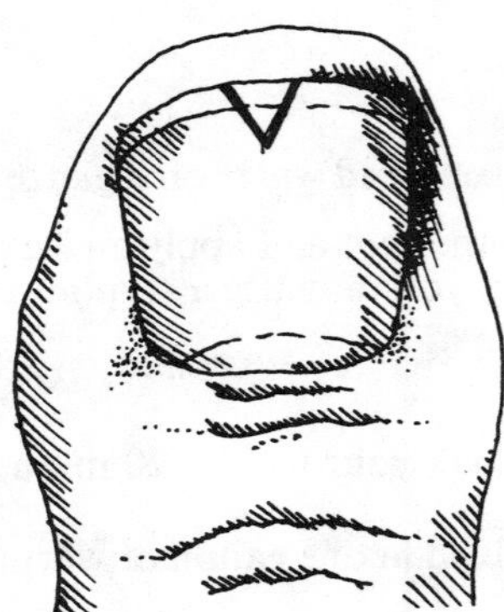

► Don't waste time cutting V's, S's, or any other design in the nail. It does not work.

► Don't use any over-the-counter preparations. They rarely work and may be dangerous.

Practical Pointers for Prevention

1. Keep your toenails clean.

2. Trim your toenails the way they are normally shaped, not necessarily straight across. Always leave the toenail a lit tle longer than you think it should be cut.

3. Watch out for excessive shoe pressure.

4. Do not wear improperly fitting shoes or socks. This advice is of particular importance for children who are used to receiving "hand-me-down" clothing and shoes from older brothers and sisters.

Chapter 4

Thick Toenail

(Onychogryphosis)

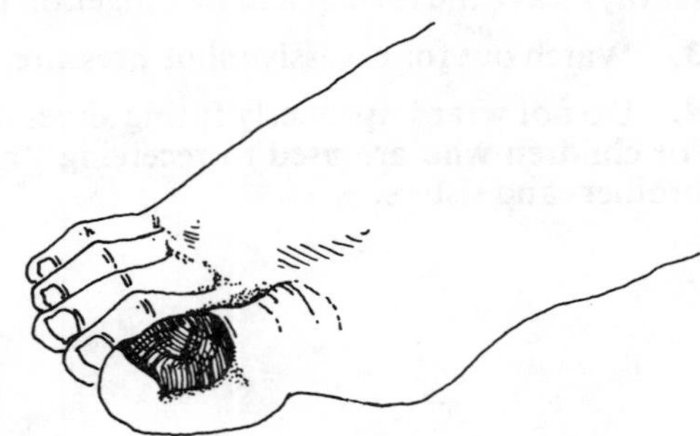

What is it?

A toenail may become thickened and/or discolored because of an injury or fungus infection. It will be dirty yellow or brown in color, with occasional blackened areas. There is usually a white or yellow crust that flakes off the toenail, and under or around the nail a cheesy substance with a strong odor may be present. The nail may be cracked and brittle. The most commonly affected nail is the large toenail.

Things you will need for this treatment

see chapter 2 "Materials List" for brand names and substitutes

ice bag
soap & water
soaking solution
antiseptic
softening agent
nail forceps-straight backed
cotton
nail file
forty percent salicylic acid plaster
nail brush
bandaids
antibiotic cream (if you have any)

Caution: ***Do not proceed with this treatment until you have read the Guidelines to Treatment in Chapter 2***

Preparation for Treatment

► Make sure any instruments you use are clean. Wash them in soap and water and rinse off with alcohol or some other recognized antiseptic.

► Make sure all materials and suggested medications are clean and up-to-date.

► Put two tablespoons of mild household detergent into ½ gallon of warm water. Dip your foot in the water and soak for 10 minutes.

► Read through all the instructions which follow, and make sure you understand them before beginning treatment.

Treatment

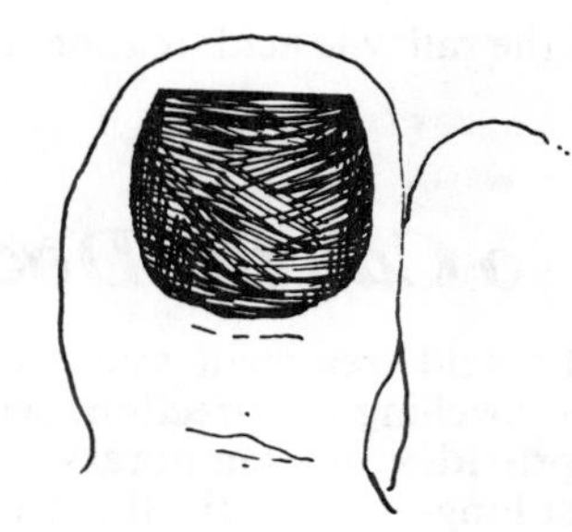

1. Cut the nail straight across with a nail nipper.

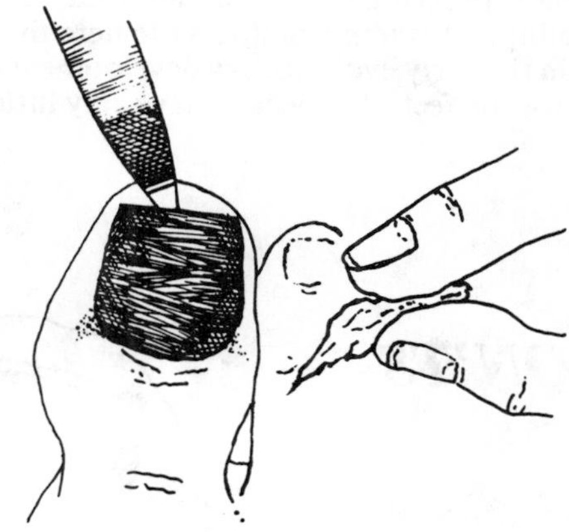

2. Take a clean nail file and a wisp of cotton, and clean out the debris under and around the sides of the toenail. You may have to do it in more than one sitting.

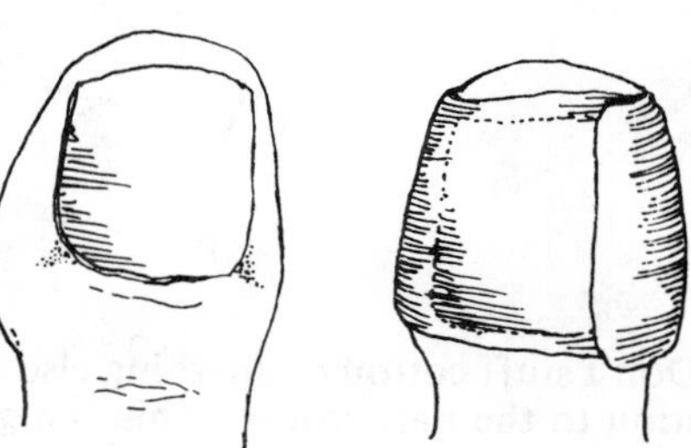

3. Cut a piece of 40% salicylic acid plaster to the size and shape of the nail plate. Put it on the nail plate with the plaster side against the nail, and cover with a bandaid. Keep the toe dry for two days.

4. When you remove the plaster, take a nail brush or an old toothbrush and brush off as much flaky nail debris as possible. Then take your nail nipper and cut as much of the nail off as you can. File down any sharp points.

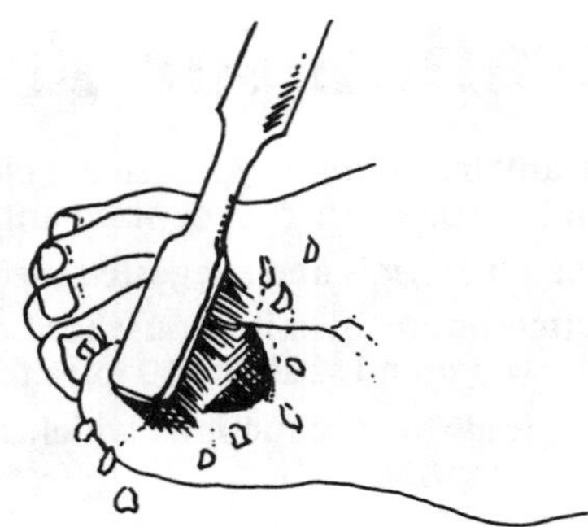

5. Thoroughly clean the area with warm, soapy water and put on an antiseptic solution like Merthiolate.

6. Repeat the salicylic acid treatment three to four times.

When to Call the Doctor

The salicylic acid treatment may cause a mild discomfort. However, if you have any severe pain, swelling or infection, see your podiatrist immediately. If the do-it-yourself treatment provides only temporary comfort and the problem soon returns, the podiatrist may suggest long-term medication therapy or permanent removal of the toenail (through a minor procedure done under local anesthetic with very little pain and almost no disability). It is important to note here that the toenails are appendages that were important in the early evolutionary development of man; but since the advent of protective shoe gear for the feet, the toenails have very little function.

DON'TS

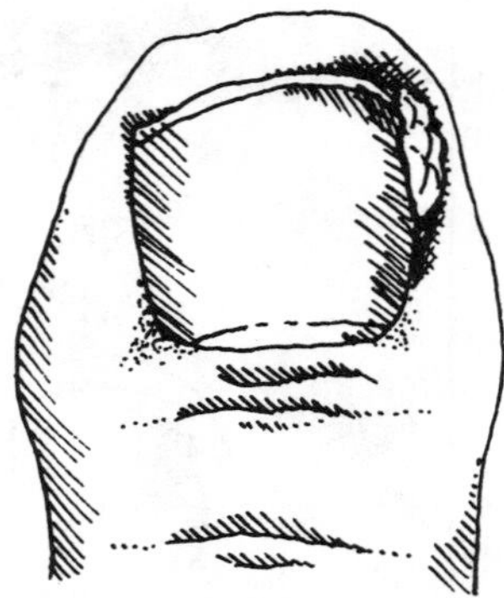

1. Don't stuff cotton or anything else under the nail edge. Cotton hardens and will cause irritation to the nail groove. This can give rise to corns in the nail groove, as well as to infection.

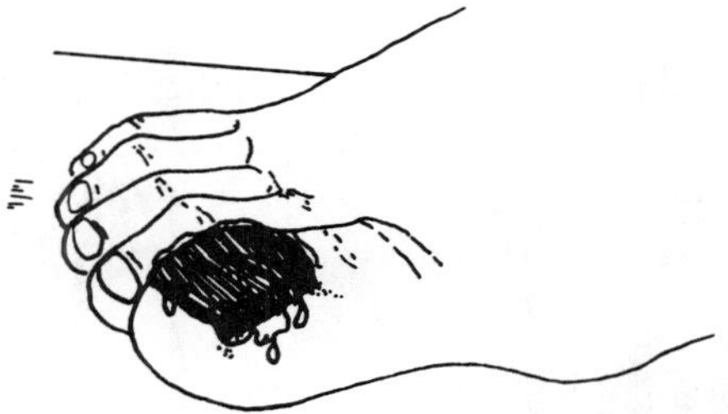

2. Don't use any over-the-counter preparations. They rarely work and may be dangerous.

Practical Pointers for Prevention

1. Keep toenails clean.

2. Watch out for excessive shoe pressure.

3. When working or doing anything where you might accidentally drop something on your toes, wear closed shoes to protect them.

4. Change shoes and socks daily, as excessive perspiration, darkness and warmth are the prerequisites for getting fungus infections of the toenails. You can't find a better environment than the inside of your shoes for creating these conditions.

Chapter 5

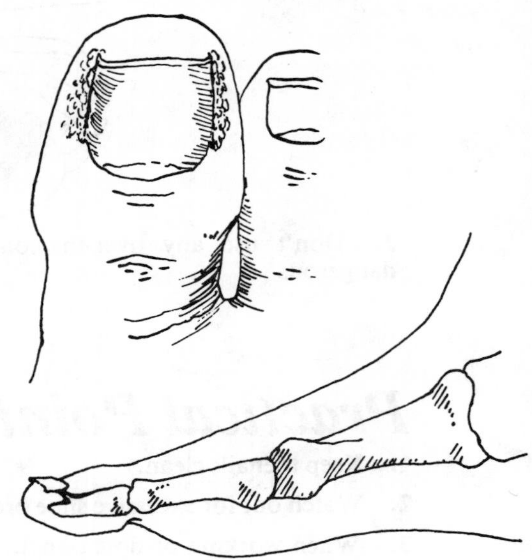

Pain Under and Around Toenail

(Subungual exostosis or calloused nail groove)

What is it?

There are two main causes of pain under and around the toenail, other than ingrown toenail (which is shown separately in Chapter 3). The two causes are (1) a bony projection, or spur, that forms on the big toe directly under the nail, resulting in painful upward pressure against the nail, and (2) a callous formation in the nail groove on either side of the nail.

Things you will need for this treatment

see chapter 2 "Materials List" for brand names and substitutes
soap & water
antiseptic
ice bag
nail forceps, straight-backed
2"x 2" gauze pads
soaking solution
bandaids
antibiotic cream (if you have any)

Caution: *Do not proceed with this treatment until you have read the Guidelines to Treatment in Chapter 2*

Preparation for Treatment

► Make sure all the materials you will be using are clean and fresh and that the forceps are clean, as discussed in chapter 2. Also make sure the foot itself is clean and dry.

► Read through all the instructions which follow, and make sure you understand them before beginning treatment.

► If you would like to numb the toe a little before beginning treatment, hold an ice pack against the toe—but not for longer than five minutes at a time.

► Put two tablespoons of mild household detergent into ½ gallon of warm water. Dip your foot in the water and soak for ten minutes.

Treatment of Callous Formation in Nail Groove

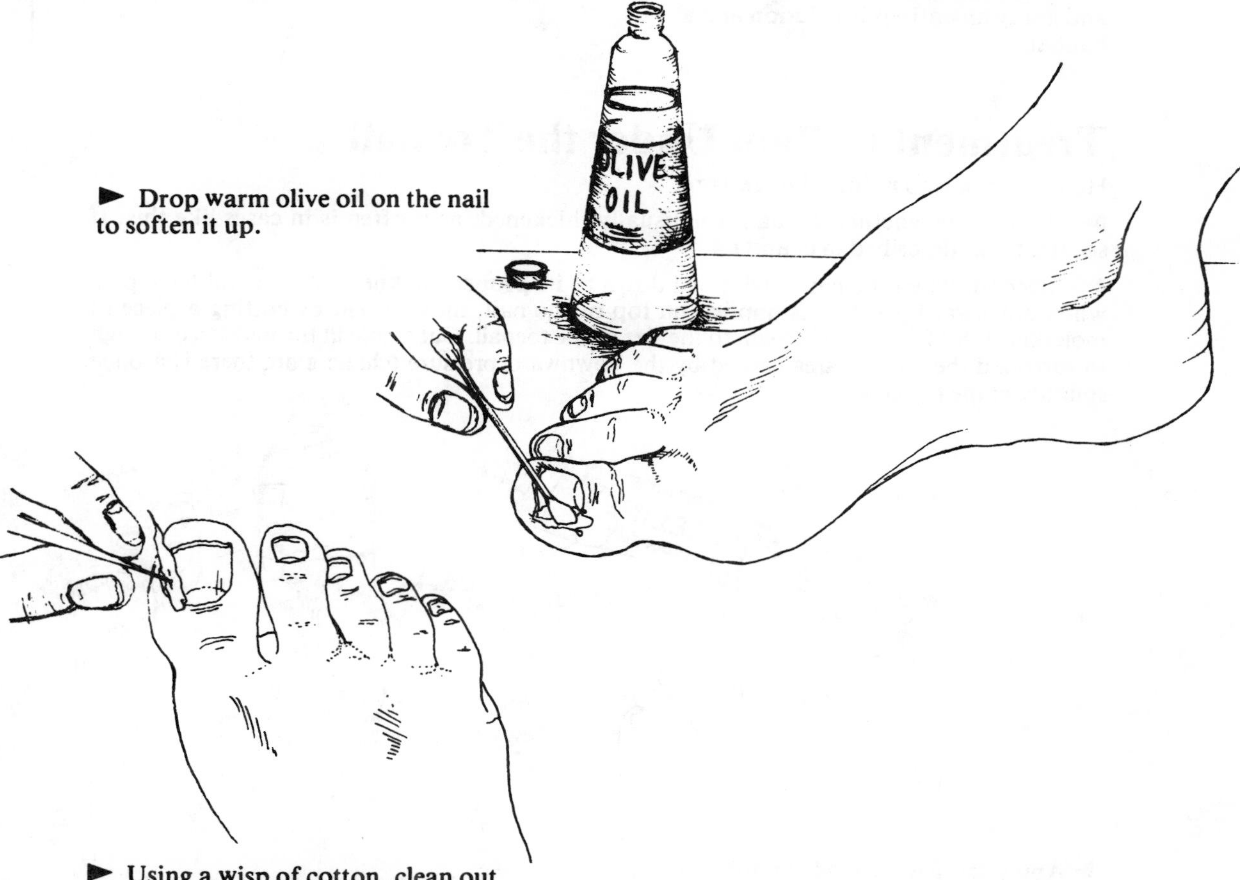

► Drop warm olive oil on the nail to soften it up.

► Using a wisp of cotton, clean out the nail groove of any soft cheesy material.

► Using forceps or tweezers, gently pull back the side of the nail groove enough to expose the callous tissue, and use the nail file to clean out the groove again.

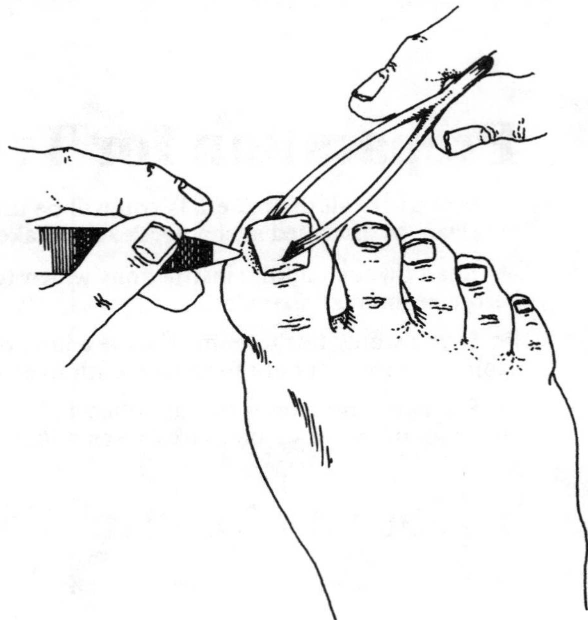

► Wash the area with soap and water and apply an antiseptic solution and a bandaid.

Treatment of Pain Under the Toenail

Here the task is to reduce the pressure.

► First, note whether the nail is unusually thickened, as it often is in cases like this. If so, treat it as described in chapter 4.

► Second, when the nail is trimmed down to its proper thickness, if you still have pain when downward pressure is applied on top of the nail, make a pad by cutting a piece of moleskin, 1/8" felt, or 1/8" foam to the size of the toenail. Cut a hole in the pad large enough to surround the painful area caused by the downward pressure (chances are there is a bone spur under the toenail).

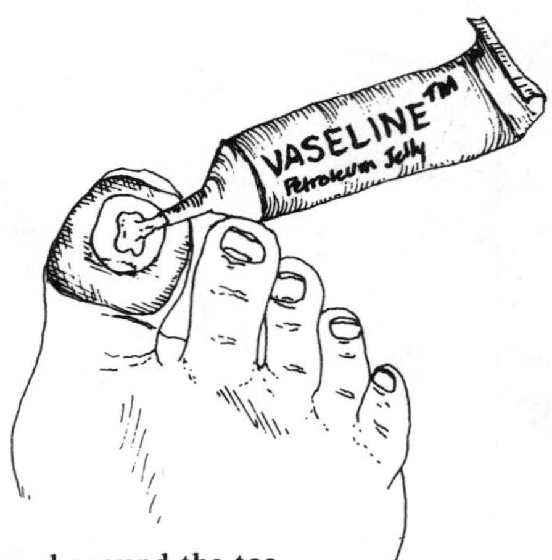

► Apply the pad around the toe. Then place a daub of VASELINE™ in the hole, and cover with a half-inch square of gauze pad.

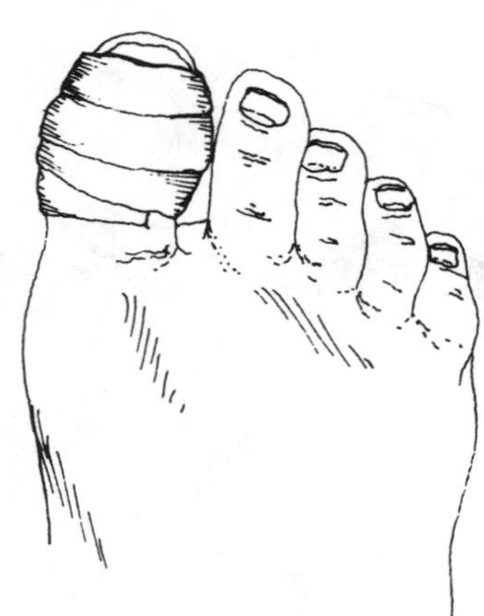

► Wrap the toe gently with bandaid or adhesive tape.

When to Call the Doctor

If pain is not reduced after one day, or if you think you have an infection (if the area is red, warm, or swollen), see a podiatrist immediately. If the do-it-yourself treatment provides only temporary comfort and the problem soon returns, you can have the callous part of the nail groove trimmed out professionally, or the pressure of a bone spur removed through a minor procedure that is done under local anesthetic with very little pain and almost no disability.

DON'TS

- Don't waste time cutting Vs in the toenail (see chapter 3)
- Don't wear narrow-toed or pointed shoes.
- Don't use over-the-counter remedies.
- Don't stuff cotton under the toenail.

Practical Pointers for Prevention

1. Avoid excessive shoe pressure.
2. Check shoes and socks for proper fit, especially pressure points or seams that could be irritating.
3. Always cut your nails as straight as possible, and do not let them dig down into the corners.

Chapter 6

Corn on Top of Toe

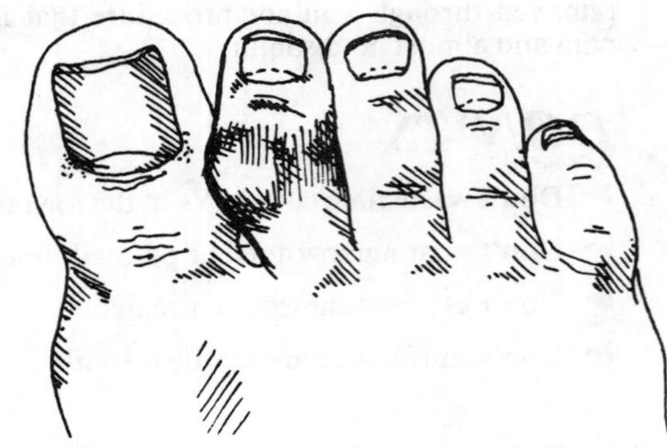

What is it?

Most corns on top of the toes are due to hammered (contracted, or claw-like) toes. The contracting usually occurs as a result of imbalances of bone structure or muscles, that make the toe stick up higher than normal and cause pressure, both from the bone inside the toe and from the shoe outside.

Things you will need for this treatment

see chapter 2 "Materials List" for brand names and substitutes

soap & water
softening agent
callous file or "mildly abrasive tool"
corn pads, non-medicated 1/8"
1/8" adhesive felt or foam or moleskin
petroleum jelly
2"x2" gauze pads
adhesive tape

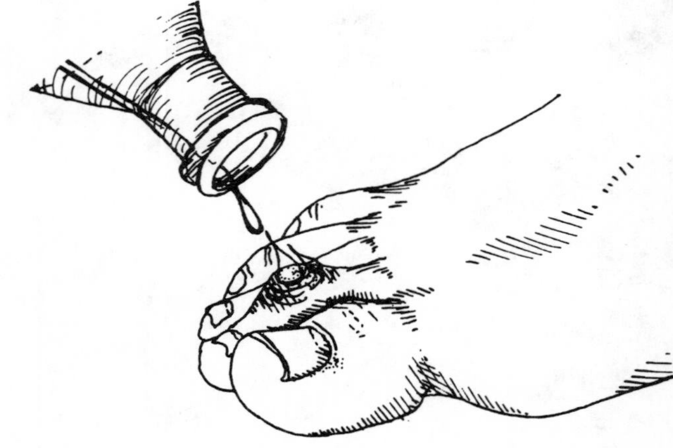

Preparation for Treatment

1. Make sure all the materials you will be using are clean and fresh as discussed in chapter 2. Also make sure the foot itself is clean and dry.

2. Read through all the instructions which follow, and make sure you understand them before beginning treatment.

3. Put two tablespoons of mild household detergent into ½-gallon of warm water. Dip your foot in the water and soak the corn for ten minutes.

4. Dry the foot and rub a few drops of cooking oil into the corn to further soften it.

Caution: *Do not proceed with this treatment until you have read the Guidelines to Treatment in Chapter 2*

Treatment

1. To provide temporary relief, remove the top layer of the corn.

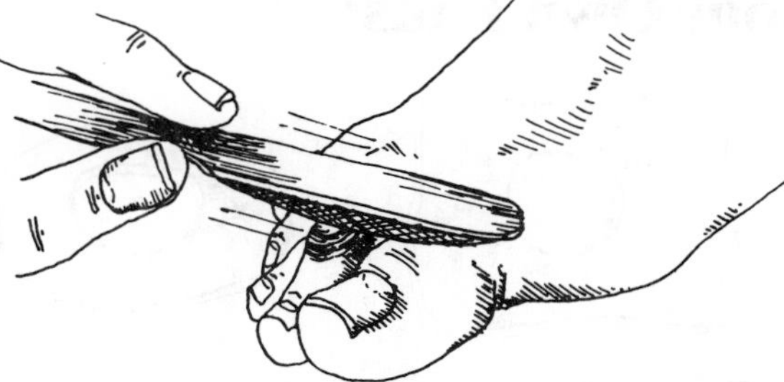

► Using a back-and-forth sawing motion, mechanically shave down the thick skin with a mildly abrasive pumice stone, sandstone, sandpaper, or callous file.

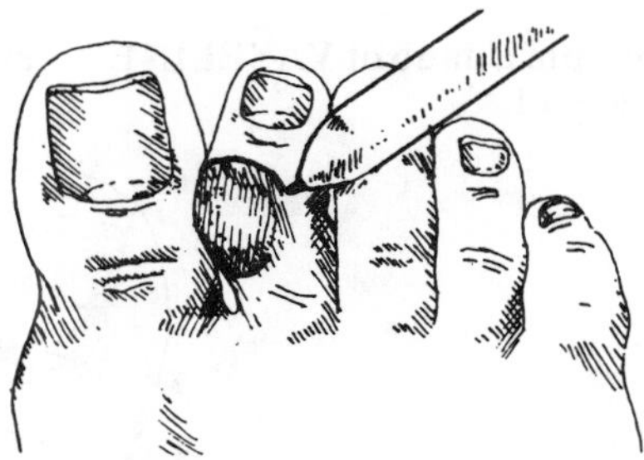

► Make sure you stay on the overlying thick skin. If you can't see the line of demarcation between the corn and the toe, it might be helpful to circle the corn with a ball point or felt tip pen.

2. After you have removed as much "top skin" as you can . . .

► Cleanse the area with soap and water, using a 2" x 2" gauze pad instead of a washcloth.

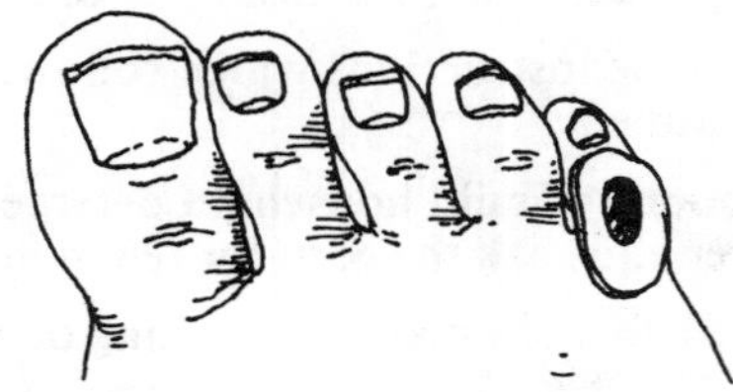

► Apply a commercially available *non-medicated* corn pad, making sure it is thick enough to cover the raised portion of the corn and that the pad overlaps the corn by at least 1/8 inch on all sides.

NOTE: To enlarge hole, gently tug from side to side and the material will usually stretch. Do this carefully, as the pad will easily tear.

To Make Your Own Pads:

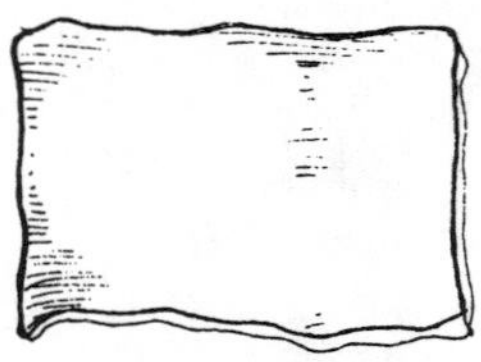

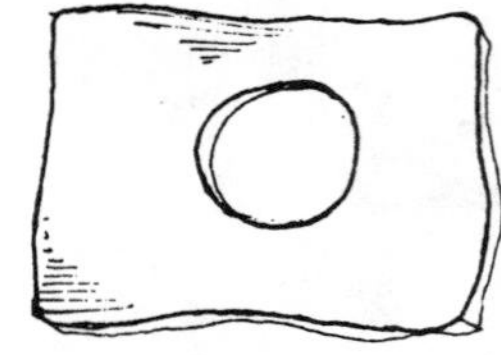

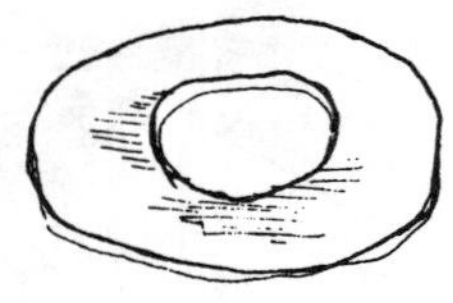

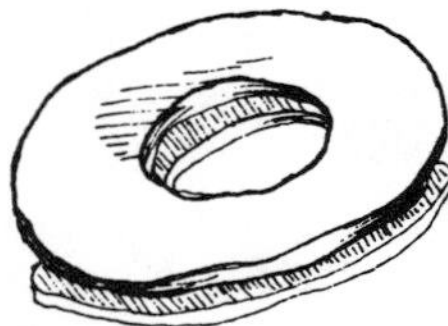

1. Take a piece of moleskin, 1/8" felt, or 1/8" foam. Cut a hole in it.

2. Trim to shape and stretch if necessary. Apply as many thicknesses as you need to remove pressure (usually one is enough).

► When the pad is in place, put a daub of VASELINE™ ointment in the hole, then cover with a ½" square of gauze pad.

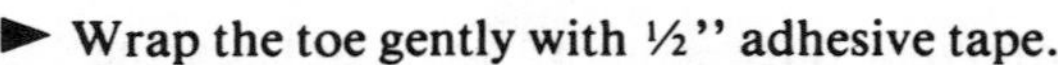

► Wrap the toe gently with ½" adhesive tape.

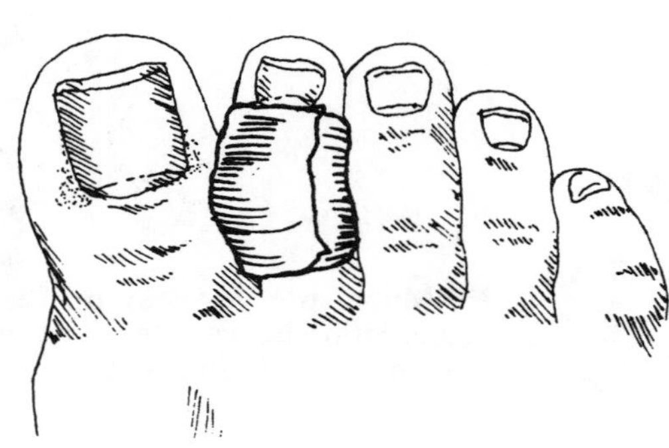

When to Call the Doctor

► If pain is not reduced in one day or you think you have an infection (if the area is red, warm, or swollen), don't touch it yourself! See a podiatrist immediately.

► This treatment provides temporary relief but does not remove the cause. Permanent correction may be available from a podiatrist, who can either keep the area trimmed down for you, or straighten the hammertoe using a procedure that causes only minor disability and has been highly successful in achieving permanent "cure" for corns of this type.

DON'TS

► Don't use razor blades

► Don't use any other sharp objects

► Don't use medicated corn pads. (They contain acids and can cause burns and infection in normal skin surrounding the corn).

► Don't put pads directly on top of a corn. This will only increase pressure and pain.

Practical Pointers for Prevention

► To relieve pressure, stretch the shoe at the spot where it covers the corn. To do this, put a broom handle into the toe box and pull the shoe downward so that the end of the handle pushes the fabric at the appropriate spot. Hold for ten minutes.

► To soften leather on new shoes, polish with Meltonian© shoe polish of proper color.

Chapter 7

Corn Between the Toes

(Heloma Molle)

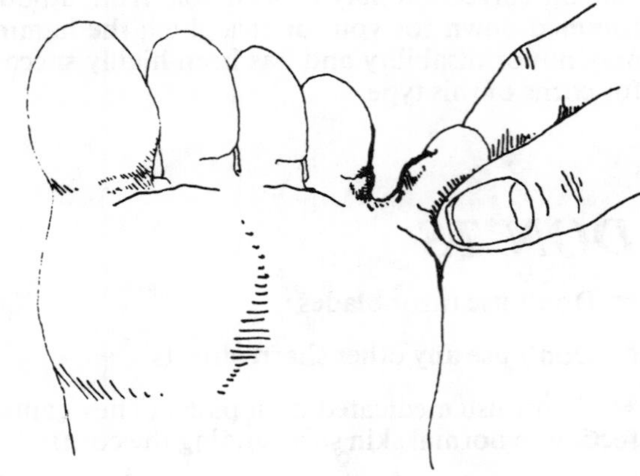

What is it?

A soft corn forms between two toes when a bony prominence in one toe becomes "attracted" to a bony prominence on the adjacent part of the toe next to it. Over a period of time, with side-to-side pressure they "hug" each other and a corn develops over each prominence. The moisture between the toes keeps the corns "soft." Initially, these soft corns must be differentiated from an early fungus infection (see chapter 14).

Things you will need for this treatment

see chapter 2 "Materials List" for brand names and substitutes

soap & water
softening agent
callous file or "mildly abrasive tool"
2"x2" gauze pads
petroleum jelly
lamb's wool

Preparation for Treatment

► Make sure any instruments you use are clean. Wash them in soap and water and rinse off with alcohol or some other recognized antiseptic.

► Make sure all materials and suggested medications are clean and up to date.

► Put two tablespoons of mild household detergent into ½ gallon of warm water. Dip your foot in the water and soak for ten minutes.

► Read through all the instructions which follow, and make sure you understand them before beginning treatment.

Caution: *Do not proceed with this treatment until you have read the Guidelines to Treatment in Chapter 2*

Treatment

1. Remove the "top layer" of the soft corn to give temporary relief.

► Make sure the corn is well-softened with oil.

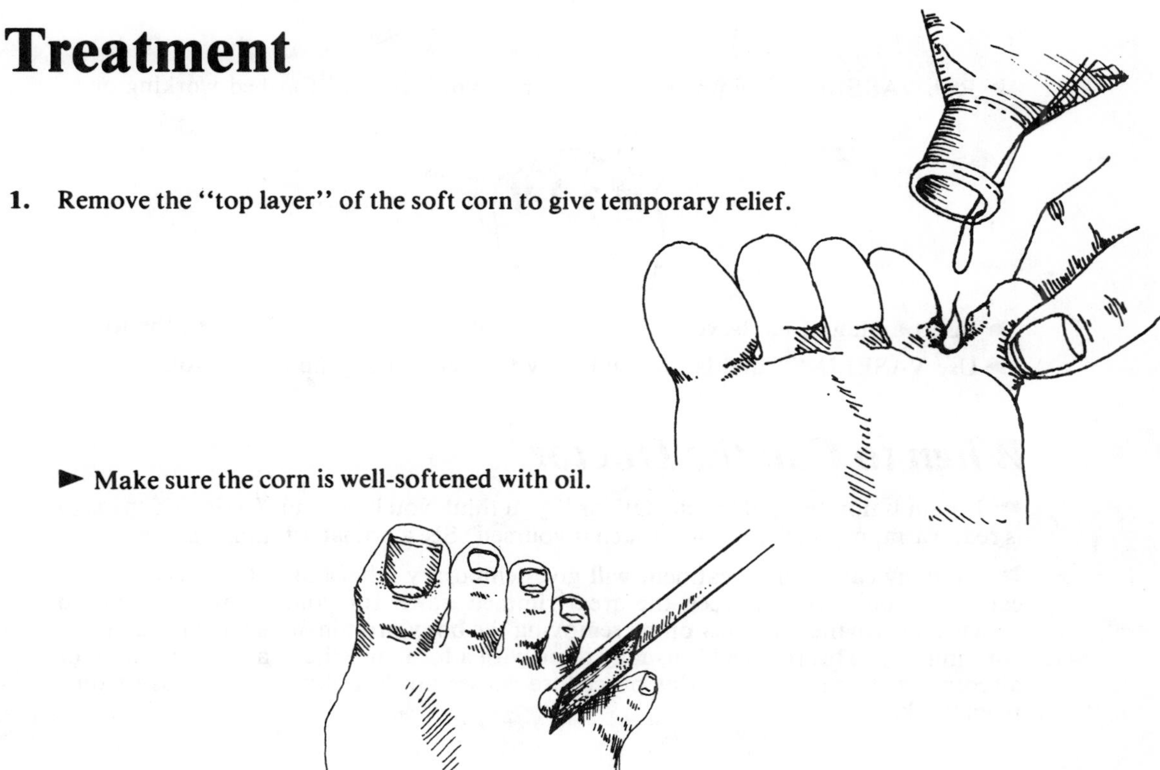

► Using your emery board or abrasive tool, file away the top layer of dead skin from the corn.

► Try to touch only the corn, keeping the abrasive tool away from the toe web (deep between the toe). If the corn is so large that it is located in the web itself, the best you can do is to skip the filing and go directly to step 2, below:

2. After you have removed as much "top skin" as you can . . .

► Cleanse the area with soap and water on a 2"x 2" gauze pad.

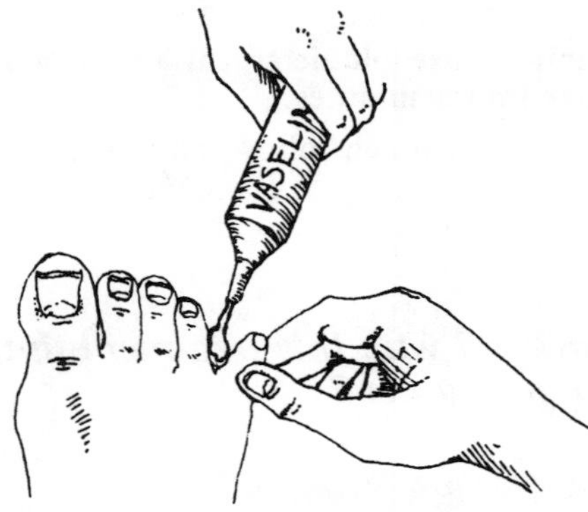

► Rub VASELINE™ ointment into the areas you have just finished working on.

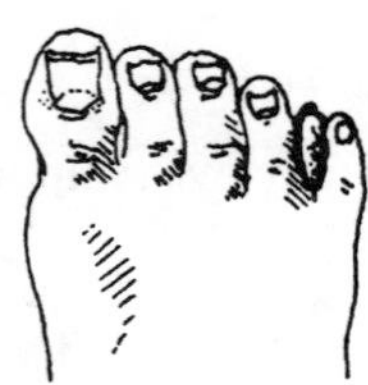

► Insert a plug of lambswool about the size of a ball of cotton between the toes.

► Use VASELINE™ and lambswool daily to keep buildup under control.

When to Call the Doctor

► If pain is not reduced in one day, or if you think you have an infection (if the area is red, warm, or swollen), don't touch it yourself! See a podiatrist immediately.

► In many cases, this treatment will give temporary relief but will not remove the cause. A podiatrist can keep the area trimmed down for you, or may be able to provide a permanent correction by removing the bony prominences which caused the corn initially. This removal is usually done with a local anesthetic and a minimum of discomfort. In many cases, this procedure causes no disability and no loss of time from work.

DON'TS

► Don't use razor blades.

► Don't use any other sharp objects.

► Don't use medicated corn pads. (They contain acids and can cause burns and infection in normal skin surrounding the corn.)

► Don't put pads directly on top of a corn. This will only increase pressure and pain.

► Don't ever stick cotton between the toes. It will harden and cause increased irritation—just the opposite of what lambswool does.

Practical Pointer for Prevention

► Make sure shoes fit properly with plenty of room for toe comfort. You should be able to freely wiggle your toes in your shoes.

How to Make Your Own Mildly Abrasive "Tool"

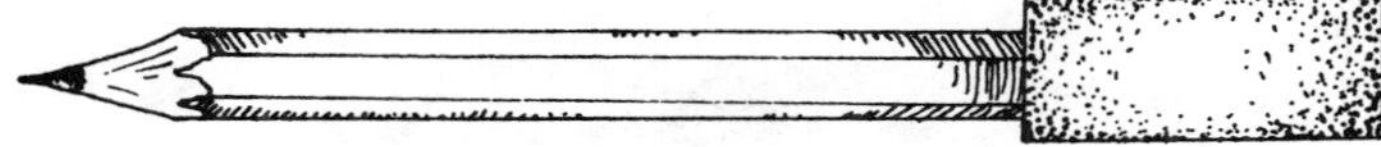

► Find a thin, clean piece of wood such as a tongue depressor, thin dowel, or a pencil.

► Glue a 1" by ½" strip of medium grade sandpaper around its end.

► Allow to dry.

Chapter 8

Callous

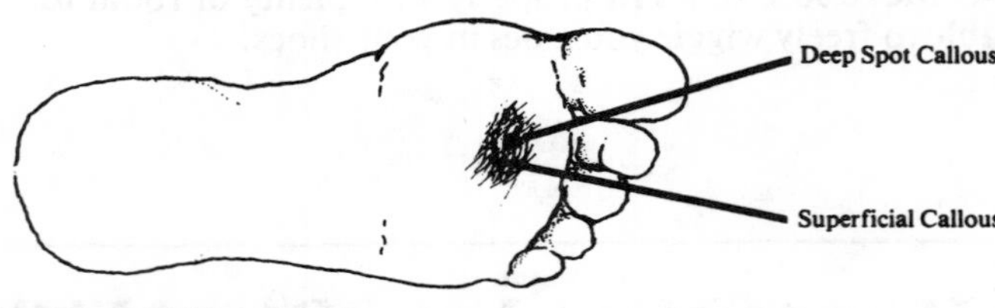

(On the Ball of the Foot)

What is it?

A callous is a buildup of thickened skin that usually occurs in areas of extreme friction and pressure—such as under the bony areas on the ball of the foot.

Usually a foot that is not aligned properly, or not mechanically sound, will "wear out" under continuous stress. What happens to the foot is like what happens when you drive a car with a poorly aligned front end, causing the tires to wear excessively in certain areas. The difference is that the foot protects itself by developing extra thickness in the skin in those spots where the skin might otherwise wear right through.

A "spot" callous is a deep, plug-like area of corny consistency located in the center of a more superficial, more spread-out callous. It is severely painful, and can cause a limp in many cases. This particular corn-within-a-callous, as it is sometimes referred to, is caused by an abnormally depressed metatarsal head, or an overlong metatarsal bone. Since all the metatarsal heads should bear an equal share of the weight load, if one is "too low" in the foot it will produce a pinpoint pressure point and a much greater stress in the skin of the bottom of the foot. You could achieve the same result from the outside-in, if you taped a pebble on the bottom of your foot and walked on it all day long!

CAUTION: If you are a diabetic or have circulatory problems, refer only to the parts of this chapter concerned with relief of pressure. It is also important to be sure that what you are treating is indeed a callous, or a corn in a callous. Sometimes a wart, an ulcer, or a foreign substance (splinter, glass, etc.) can resemble a deep callous in appearance and symptoms.

Things you will need for this treatment

see chapter 2 "Materials List" for brand names and substitutes

soaking solution
softening agent
callous file
moleskin
petroleum jelly
adhesive tape
2"x2" gauze pad
adhesive spray and skin protectant
adhesive foam or felt 1/8"

Caution: ***Do not proceed with this treatment until you have read the Guidelines to Treatment in Chapter 2***

Preparation for Treatment

► Make sure all materials and suggested medications are clean and up to date.

► Thoroughly scrub the entire foot with warm soapy water and a terry wash cloth. Pat dry with a soft clean towel.

► Read through all instructions that follow, and make sure you understand them before beginning treatment.

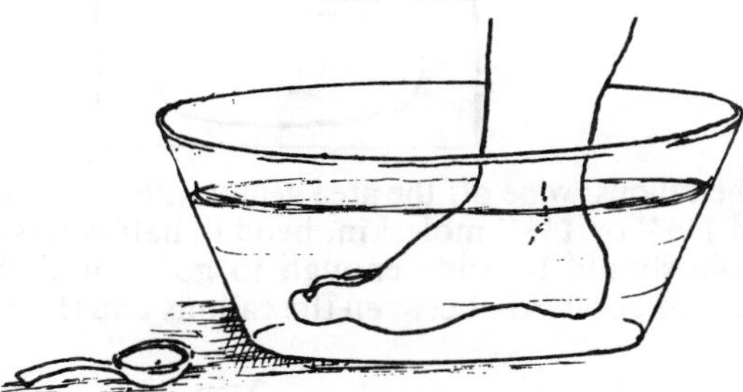

► Put two tablespoons of mild household detergent into half a gallon of warm water. Soak for twenty minutes.

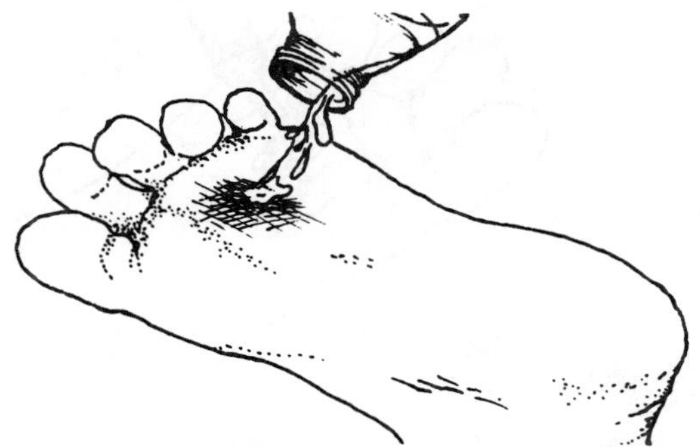

► Rub about 5 drops of cooking oil into the callous to soften it further.

Treatment

The same *general* treatment is recommended for all types of callous, but a few special suggestions will be given for each of the different types discussed in this book.

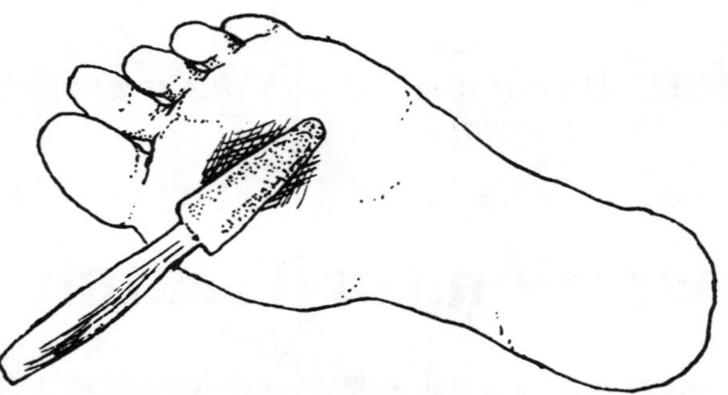

1. **Filing down the callous.**
► Using a back and forth sawing motion, remove the thick skin with a pumice stone, sandstone, mildly abrasive sandpaper, or callous file.
► Make sure you stay on the thickened skin.

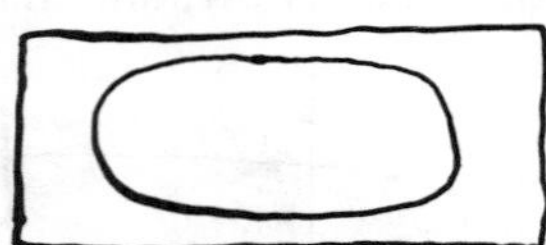

2. After filing down the callous, wipe off the area gently with soap and water on a gauze pad.
► Take a piece of 1½'' by 1½'' moleskin, bend in half with sticky side up, and cut a hole in it. The hole should be wide enough to go around the filed-down callous, leaving 1/8'' border of good skin between the callous and the pad.

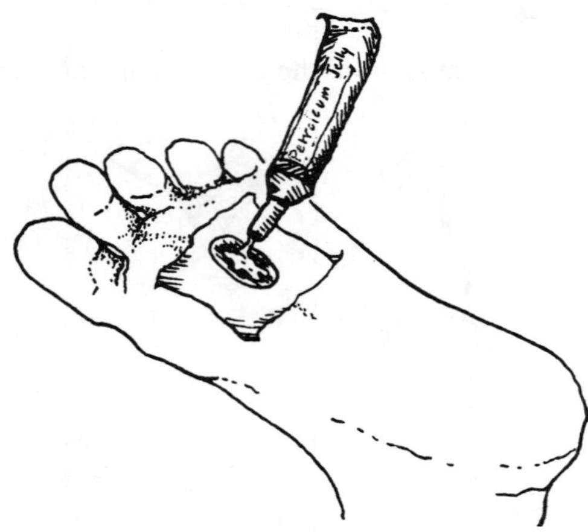

3. After the pad is properly placed on the foot, plase VASELINE™ in the hole.

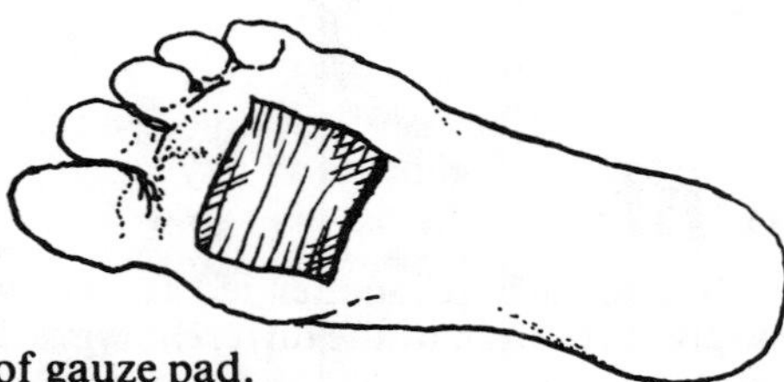

► Cover with a ½'' square of gauze pad.
► Cover this with a strip of 1'' adhesive tape.

4. Once you have trimmed and medicated the callous, it is very important to pad pressure away from it. You will need the following additional materials: A "stick'em," such as tincture of Benzoin; 1/8" foam or felt.

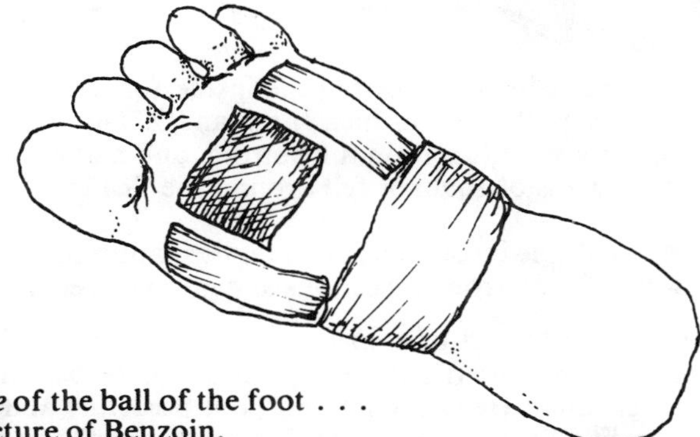

If your callous is in the *middle* of the ball of the foot . . .

► Prepare area with tincture of Benzoin.
► Cut 2 strips of foam or felt ½" wide and 2" long.
► Cut 1 strip 2" wide by 2" long.

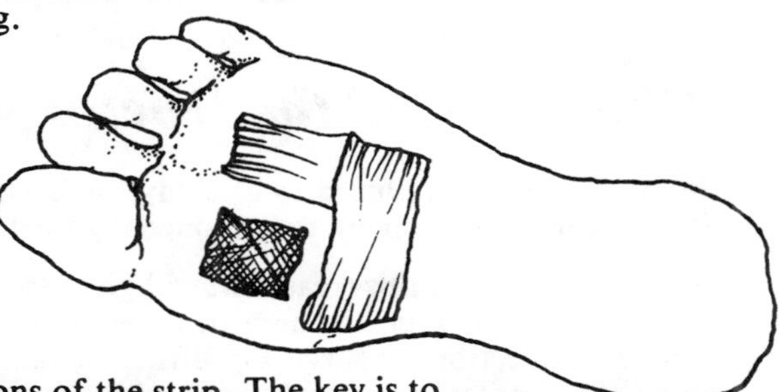

For isolated callouses, use combinations of the strip. The key is to redistribute the weight of the body away from the painful callous.

NOTE: For treatment of the heel, no pads are used. Heel callous is discussed separately (see chapter 9).

5. Keep pads completely dry for one full day, after which it is OK to get them wet. We don't recommend total saturation with wetness, however. Don't swim or take baths, and confine your bathing to quick showers as long as the pads are on. You may use a hair dryer to blow them dry after your shower.

► After wearing these pads for five days, *carefully* remove them by pulling tape from the toes toward your heel. To avoid pulling skin off the foot, peel very slowly and gently (see chapter 2).

► Apply powder liberally when dry.

NOTE: If you are allergic to adhesive tape, ask your druggist for non-allergenic paper tape.

6. For longer relief between home treatments, you can make a balanced inlay for your shoes to keep pressure off your callouses all day long.

► Go to a drug store or athletic shoe shop and pick up a pair of Dr. Scholl's full length foam rubber insoles or Spenco insoles.

► Wear them for one week, and your callouses will leave impressions on the insole, locating the areas of greatest stress and showing you the spots *around which* the insole needs to be built up to even out the pressure.

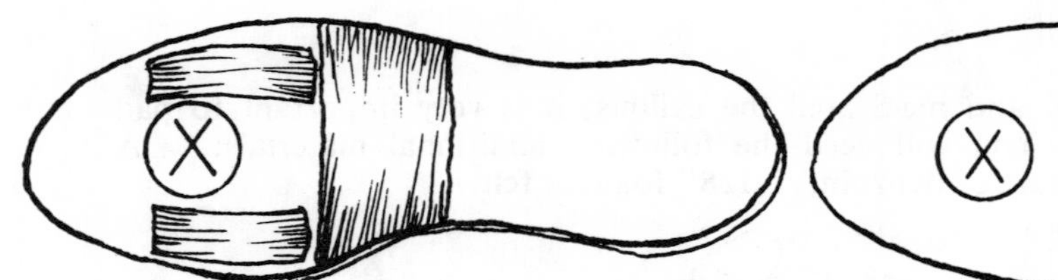
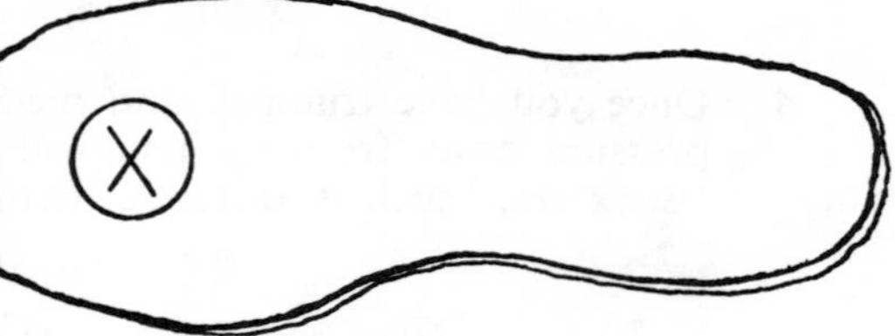

► Or, instead of wearing the insole for a week, try holding it against your foot to feel where the callous hits. Mark an "X" at the spot. Push in hard on that "X" until you feel your finger on the bottom, and make a large circle around your finger. Glue your strips of foam or felt around the "callous" area (circle) just as you did on your foot.

► With the insole in your shoe, the pads underneath the insole will redistribute your weight away from the callous and give you relief.

If you are flatfooted or pronate (roll foot from the outside inward) excessively, you will probably have more friction and pressure on the ball of your foot—and may be more likely to have callouses (see appendix on Foot Structure and Function). To reduce this excessive pressure, fit a Spenco inlay to your shoe and attach to it a varus wedge long enough to extend from the heel to the arch (see appendix on Shoe Inserts You Can Make).

When to Call the Doctor

► If pain is not reduced in one day, or if you think you have an infection (if the area is red, warm, or swollen), don't touch it yourself! See a podiatrist immediately.

► In many cases, this treatment will give temporary relief but will not remove the cause. A podiatrist can keep the area trimmed down for you, or may be able to provide a permanent correction by surgically lifting the abnormally depressed or overlong matatarsal bone. This removal is usually done with a local anesthetic and a minimum of discomfort. In many cases, this procedure causes no disability and no loss of time from work.

To make your own callous file:

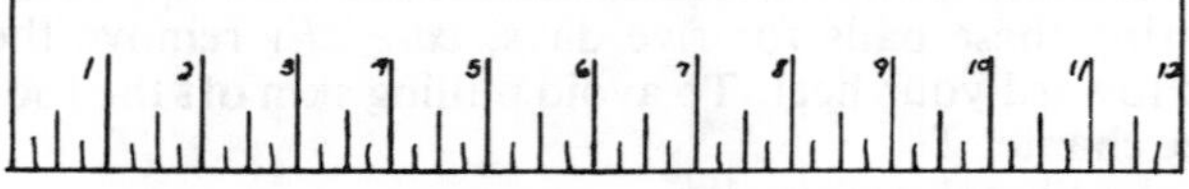

1. Take a one-foot wooden ruler (or any similar smooth-finished piece of wood)...

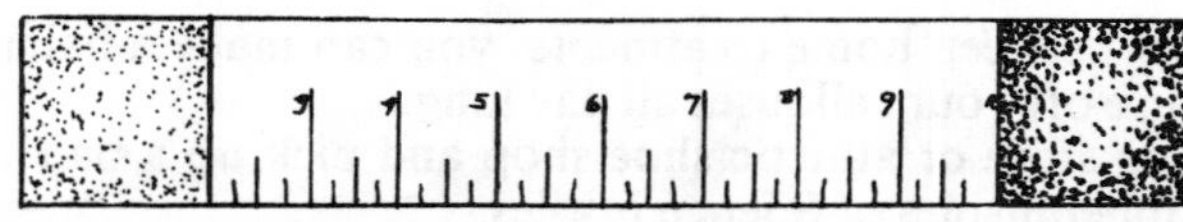

2. Glue a 2″ × 2″ piece of mildly abrasive grade sandpaper on one end and a 2″ × 2″ piece of "fine" sandpaper on the other end.
3. Begin treatment using mildly abrasive paper and finish with fine paper.

Chapter 9

Heel Callous and Fissures

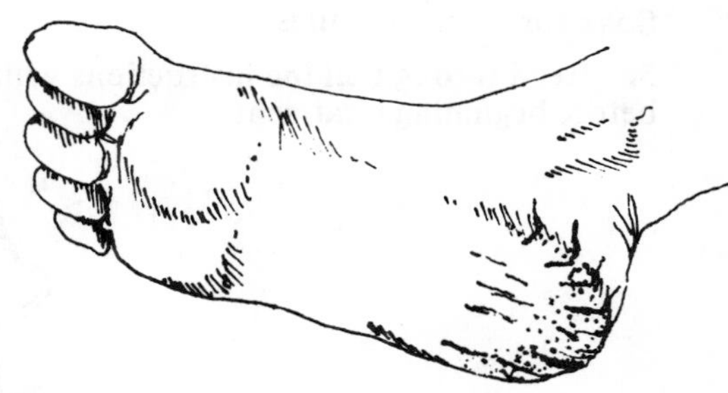

What is it?

A heel callous is a build-up of thickened skin caused by excessive friction between the skin of the heel and the sock or shoe. For example, a foot that is not properly aligned causes excessive movement of the heel bone against the shoe. When this happens, the skin which is caught between the bone and leather has to thicken to protect itself from irritation. Open backed sandals, slingback shoes, and "mule" type step-in shoes and slippers can aggravate this problem by slapping against the heel with each step and moving in the opposite direction of the foot. This causes especially rapid build-up of callous. Thick callouses will sometimes crack and split through to the uncalloused skin. These deep cracks, or fissures, may bleed and become quite painful. If not treated, they may even become infected.

Things you will need for this treatment

see chapter 2 "Materials List" for brand names and substitutes

soap & water
soaking solution
softening agent
callous file or "mildly abrasive tool"
petroleum jelly
heel cups
medicated foot powder

Caution: ***Do not proceed with this treatment until you have read the Guidelines to Treatment in Chapter 2***

Preparation for Treatment

1. Make sure all the materials you will be using are clean and fresh as discussed in chapter 2.

2. Put two tablespoonfuls of mild household detergent into a half gallon of warm water. Soak for twenty minutes.

3. Read through all the instructions which follow, and make sure you understand them before beginning treatment.

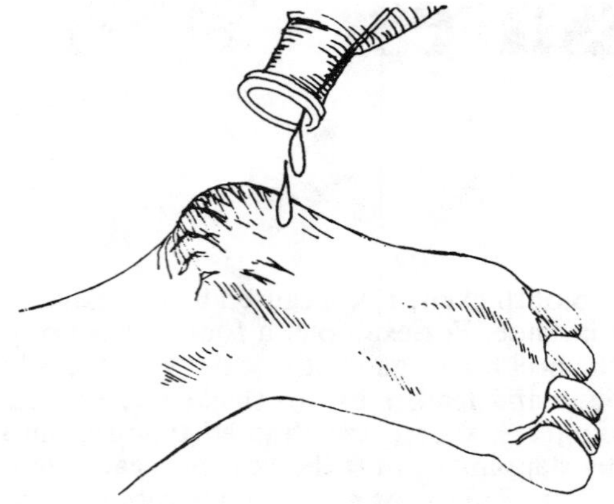

5. Rub about 5 drops of cooking oil into the callous to soften it further.

Treatment

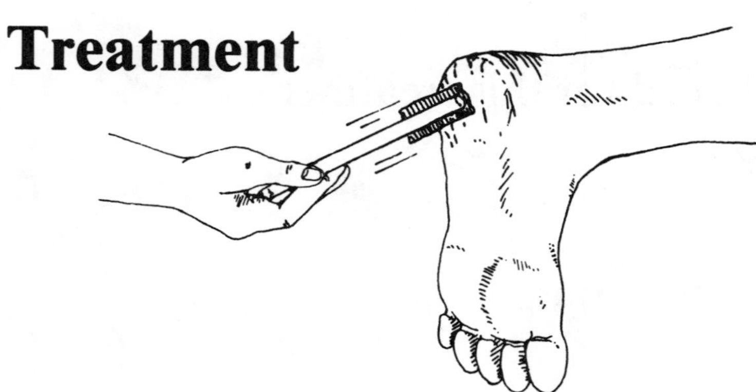

► Using a back-and-forth sawing motion, remove the thick skin with a pumice stone, mildly abrasive sandpaper, or callous file. (You can make your own file by gluing sandpaper to a wooden ruler (see chapter 8).

During the next two weeks . . .

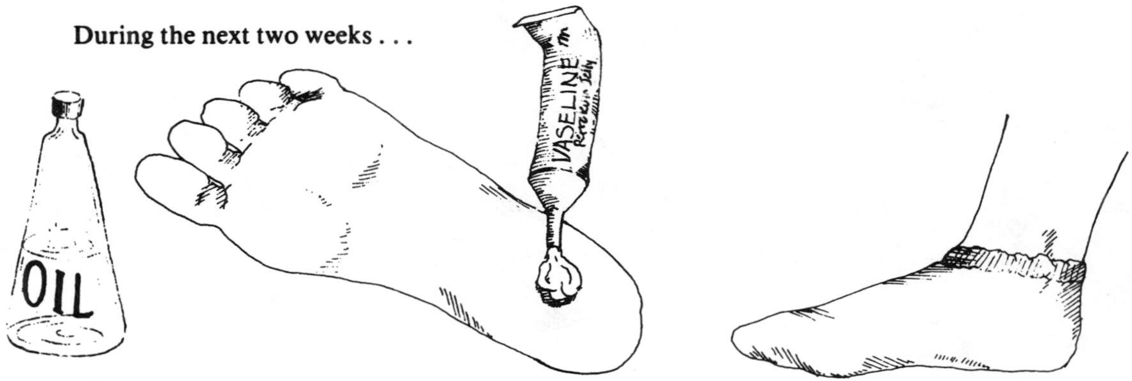

► Before going to bed, rub in some cooking oil, cover with VASELINE,™ and put on a pair of white cotton socks for the night.

► Continue this procedure for two weeks.

► After two weeks, repeat this procedure once a week for two or three more weeks.

If you are a runner or weekend athlete:

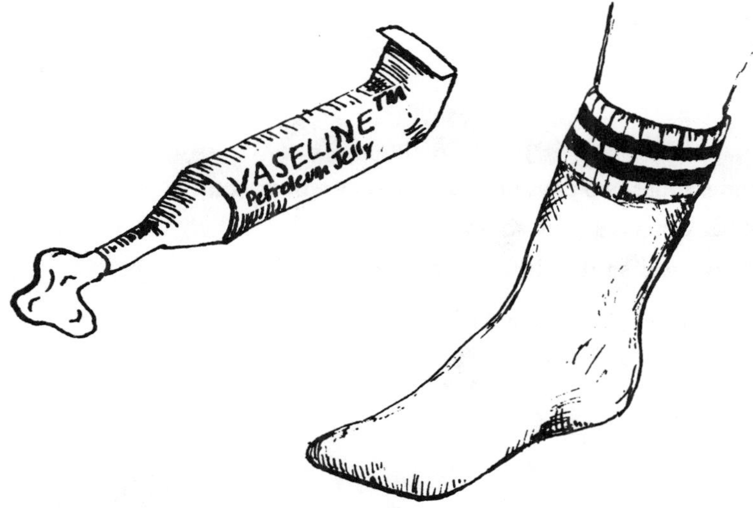

► Coat the area with VASELINE™ before running.

► Put a "ped" on the foot, and a cotton sock over the ped.

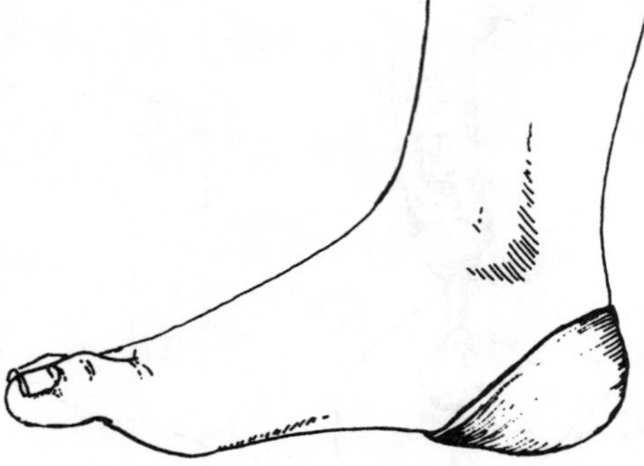

► Try using a heel cup (available in drug and sporting goods stores).

When to Call the Doctor

If you have tried the recommended treatment for several weeks and the condition is still present, or if the heel is red and hot, you need professional care.

DON'TS

► Don't wear the same shoes two days in a row, so they will dry out.

► Don't wear open back or sling back shoes.

► Don't go barefoot or wear shoes without socks.

► If you perspire excessively, see chapter 13.

Chapter 10

Warts

(Plantar verruca)

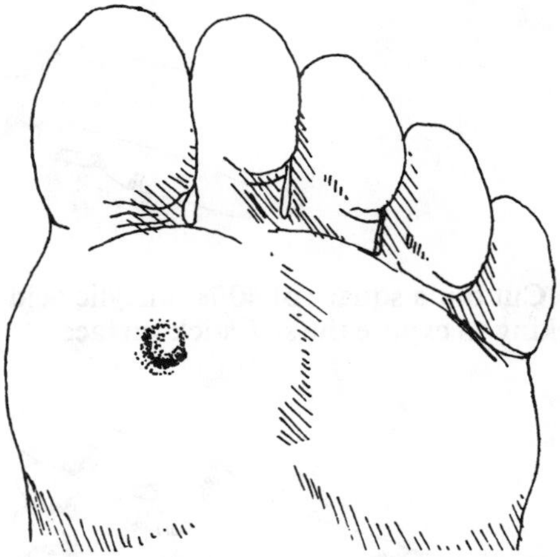

What is it?

A wart is a virus infection that can occur anywhere on the body. It usually looks a little like a tiny cauliflower projecting from the skin, except when it occurs on the bottom of the foot. Then, due to the constant weight of the body, the wart grows "into" the foot instead of "out" of it. Although warts are sometimes confused with corns and callouses, if you look at them closely you can see a well-defined border and little dark spots resembling blood vessels running all through them. They are also more sensitive to side-to-side pressure, while corns are more sensitive to direct pressure. Warts occur both singly and in clusters. They are contagious, and are especially prevalent in the fall and spring. Children are more susceptible than adults.

Things you will need for this treatment

see chapter 2 "Materials List" for brand names and substitutes

soap & water
scissors
40% salicylic acid plaster
toothbrush
bandaid or adhesive tape

Caution: *Do not proceed with this treatment until you have read the Guidelines to Treatment in Chapter 2*

Preparation for Treatment

► Make sure all the materials you will be using are clean and fresh as discussed in chapter 2.

► Put two tablespoons of mild household detergent into ½ gallon of warm water. Dip your foot in the water and soak for ten minutes.

► Read through all the instructions which follow, and make sure you understand them before beginning treatment.

Treatment

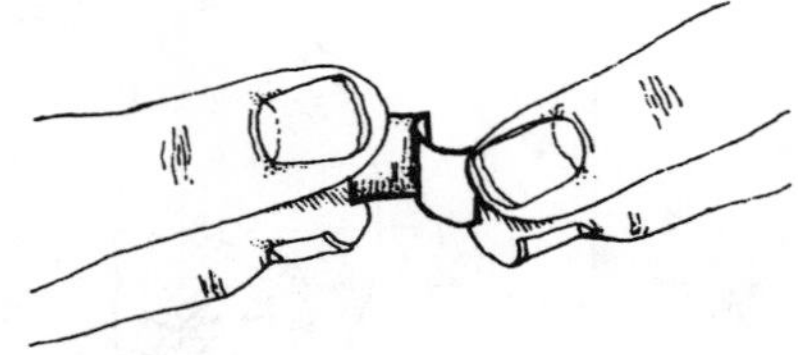

1. Cut out a square of 40% salicylic acid plaster (about the size of the wart) and remove backing to expose the self-stick surface.

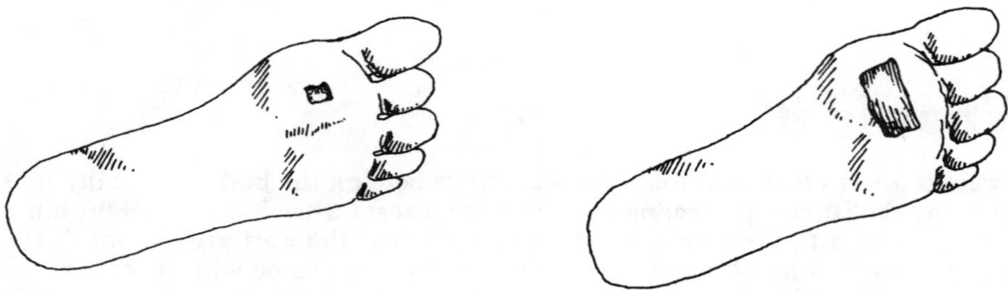

2. Apply sticky side directly onto the wart. Push down and cover with bandaid or tape.

3. For the next two days . . .
► Keep the plaster on and dry

4. After two days . . .

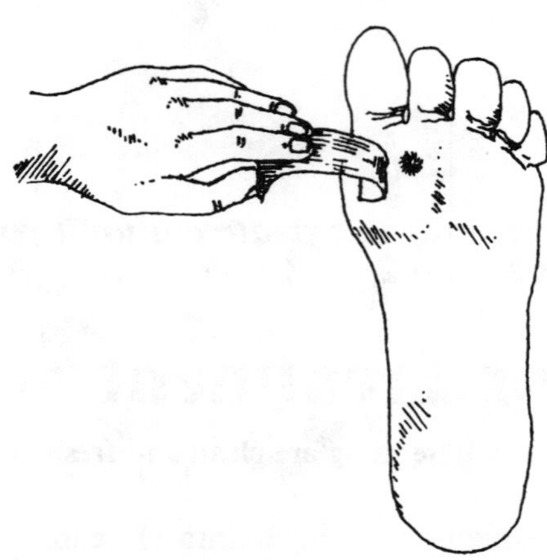

► Carefully remove the bandaid, tape and plaster. The wart will have a whitish appearance.

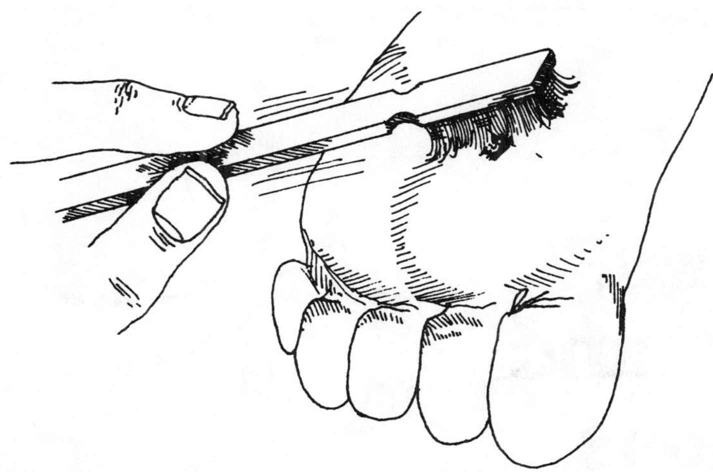

► Using the toothbrush and a little soap and water, brush the wart vigorously for one minute twice a day for two days.
► Expose the wart to the air as much as possible.

5. Repeat the entire process—two days of plaster followed by two days of brushing—for a period of two weeks.

When to Call the Doctor

If there is no improvement, or if the pain increases or the wart or warts spread, see your podiatrist. He will either treat it over a period of several weeks with different medications, or remove it by using a minor procedure that results in very little pain and only slight temporary disability.

DON'TS

► Don't use razor blades, knives or any other sharp objects on the wart!

► Don't use any drug store remedies except as directed here.

► Don't let the salicylic acid touch "normal" skin, if you can help it.

Practical Pointers for Prevention

1. Do not go barefoot.

2. Change shoes every day. Do not wear the same shoes daily.

3. If your feet perspire excessively, you may be prone to warts (see chapter 13).

4. Children are prone to this condition. Check their feet periodically, especially during fall and spring months. Early treatment is a good prevention for spread and contagiousness.

Chapter 11

Needles, Glass, and Splinters

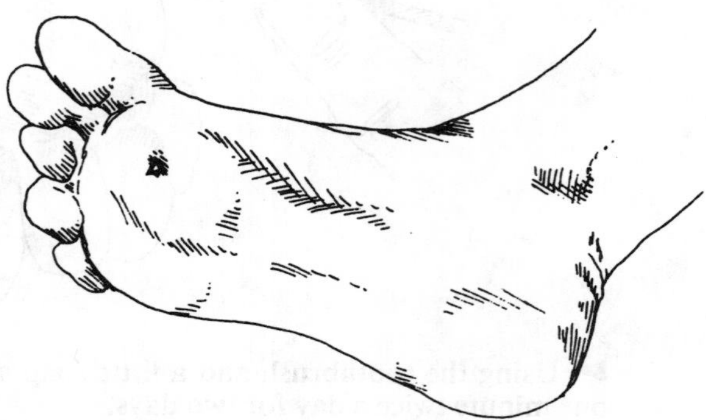

This treatment can be used whenever a foreign body becomes imbedded in the foot. A "foreign body" is anything that gets stuck in the foot and doesn't belong there—most often, a splinter of wood or a sliver of glass.

Things you will need for this treatment

see chapter 2 "Materials List" for brand names and substitutes

soap & water
antiseptic
ice bag
softening agent
2"x2" gauze pads
soaking solution
bandaid
antibiotic cream (if you have any)
pin, needle or tweezers
match

***Caution:* Do not proceed with this treatment until you have read the Guidelines to Treatment in Chapter 2**

Treatment

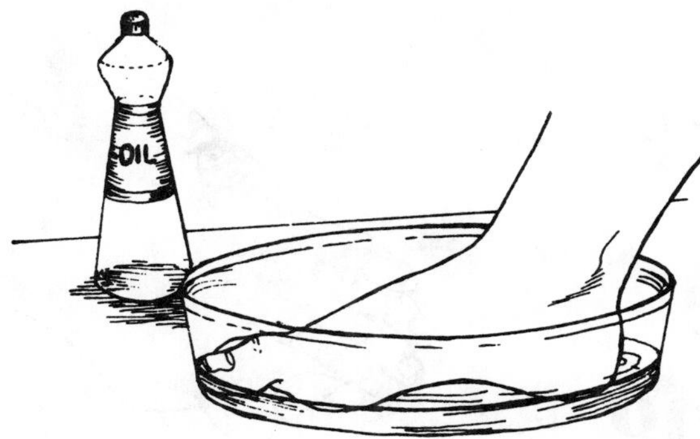

1. Soak the injured part in vegetable oil for a few minutes.

2. Apply ice to the area for 6-12 minutes, until numb.

3. Sterilize a pin, needle, or tweezers, by putting the tip into a flame of a match or dipping it in alcohol.

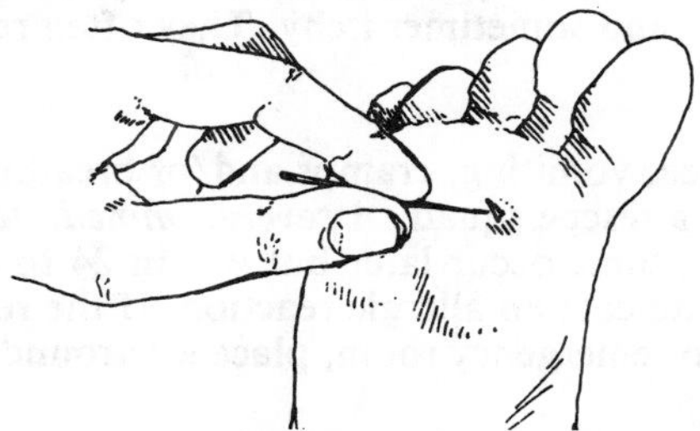

4. Use the pin to try to move the foreign body out. After soaking in oil, the foreign body should be loose and easy to remove.

5. Once the foreign body is removed, clean the area with soap and water and dry with gauze pads.

6. Apply Merthiolate or antibiotic cream and cover with a bandaid.

7. Once a day for two weeks, soak the injured part in a solution of Domeboro or epsom salts.

When to Call the Doctor

If there is any persistent redness, swelling, or drainage from the area, or if you can't remove the object yourself, see a podiatrist immediately.

NOTE: If you can't easily get to the injured area of your foot, have someone else follow these instructions for you.

Chapter 12

Bee Sting

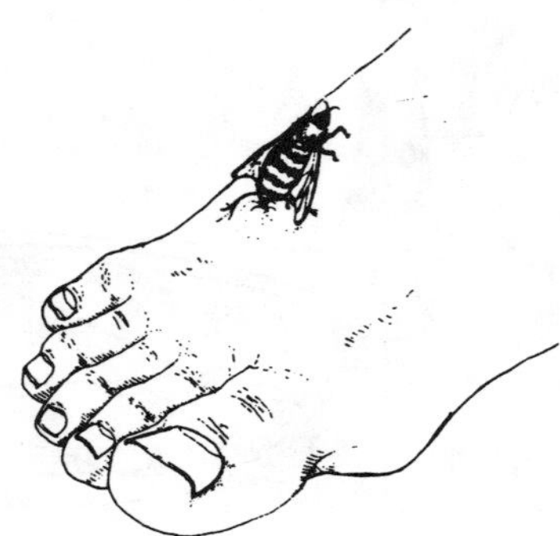

In most cases, the stings of bees and other insects are not very serious. In many cases, no treatment is necessary. However, for people who are allergic to bee stings, treatment is of urgent importance. This type of allergic reaction is usually caused by the sting of a bumble bee, hornet, wasp, or yellow jacket. It may also be caused by the bite from an ant or spider. Stings are usually painful, and sometimes itchy. They often result in swelling and heat.

CAUTION: If chills, fever, nausea, vomiting, cramps and/or breathing difficulties occur within minutes after a sting, call a rescue squad. *A severe, immediate reaction signifies a medical emergency.* If these symptoms occur later but within 24 to 48 hours, contact a doctor. Such symptoms usually indicate an allergic reaction. If the reaction is severe and you are on your way to a doctor or emergency room, place ice around the area to slow the absorption of venom.

If the reaction is localized, swelling and itching due to multiple bites in an area might last 24 to 48 hours before starting to subside. If you show any unusual allergic reaction at all to your very first sting, stay away from areas where these insects are prevalent and make proper arrangements with your physician for the handling of any future sting.

Things you will need for this treatment

see chapter 2 "Materials List" for brand names and substitutes

soap & water
ice bag
softening agent
pin, needle or tweezers
desensitizing lotion

Caution: *Do not proceed with this treatment until you have read the Guidelines to Treatment in Chapter 2*

Treatment

1. Put ice on the area for 15 to 30 minutes to numb it and help reduce the swelling.
2. Wash the area with soap and water.

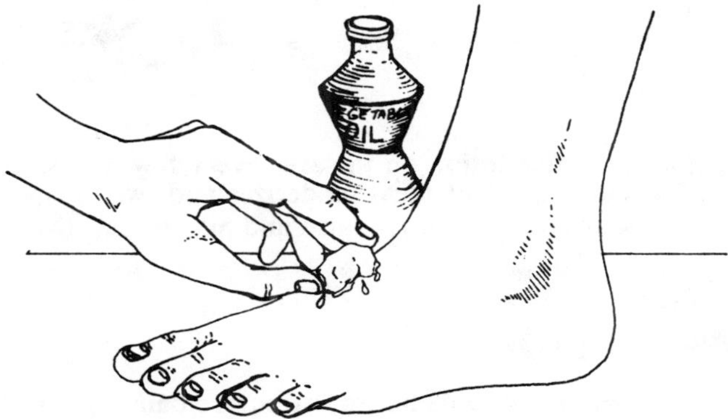

3. Coat the wound with vegetable oil for about thirty minutes.

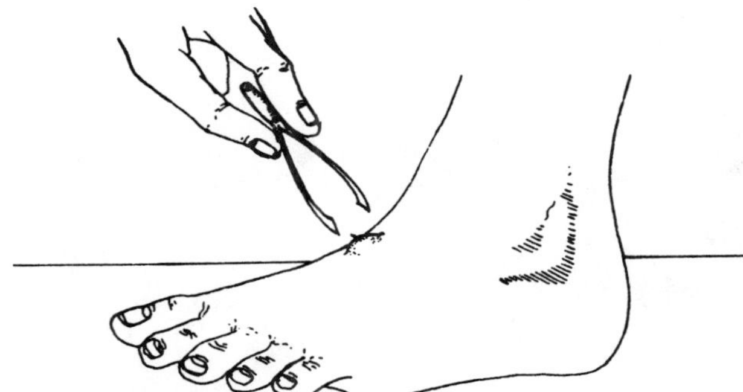

4. If a stinger is visible in the wound, try to remove it with sterilized tweezers.
5. Repeat the ice treatment (or soak in cold water) for about 15 minutes.

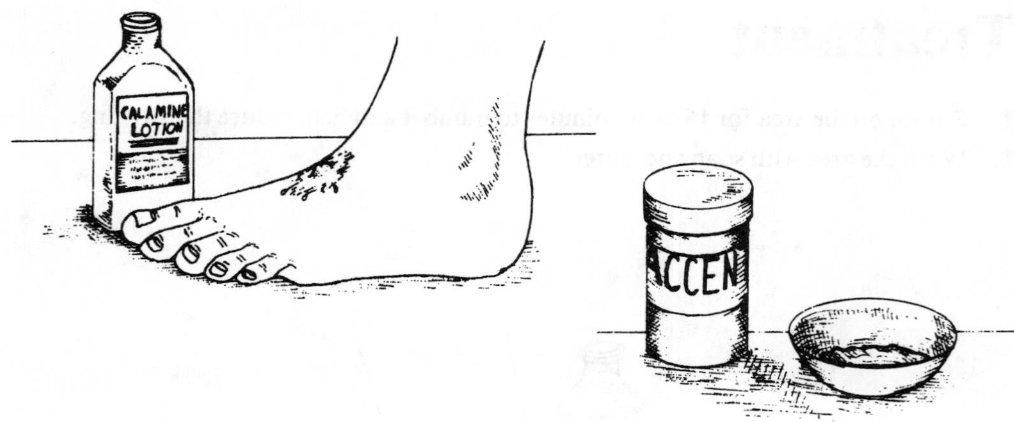

6. **If there is any itching, put Calamine lotion on the area every few hours, or make a homemade paste out of half a teaspoonful of meat tenderizer and two teaspoonfuls of water, and place on the area. Baking soda is effective also and may be substituted for the meat tenderizer.**

When to Call the Doctor

If the swelling does not go down within 24 to 48 hours and severe pain remains (or if the stinger cannot be removed), consult a podiatrist. If you can't do this treatment yourself, have someone else follow the instructions and do it for you.

Chapter 13

Sweaty and Smelly Feet

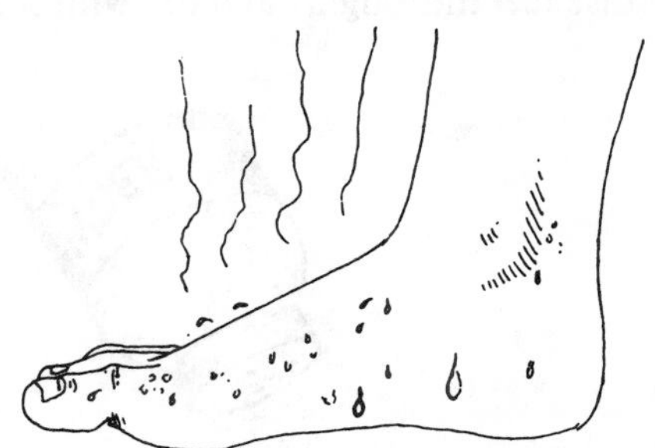

(Hyperhidrosis and Bromhidrosis)

Excessive perspiration occurs when feet sweat too much due to overactivity of the sweat glands. It is a common problem for children and young adults.

The problem of smelly feet—not "normally" smelly feet, but those with an unusually foul odor—is usually caused either by bacteria which decompose skin by-products, or by localized fungus infections (see chapter 14). The problem of odor is especially common in feet that perspire excessively.

Things you will need for this treatment

see chapter 2 "Materials List" for brand names and substitutes

soap & water
fabric for removal of dead skin
medicated foot powder
disinfectant spray
material to inhibit odor
antiperspirant
occlusive wrap
cotton swab

Treatment

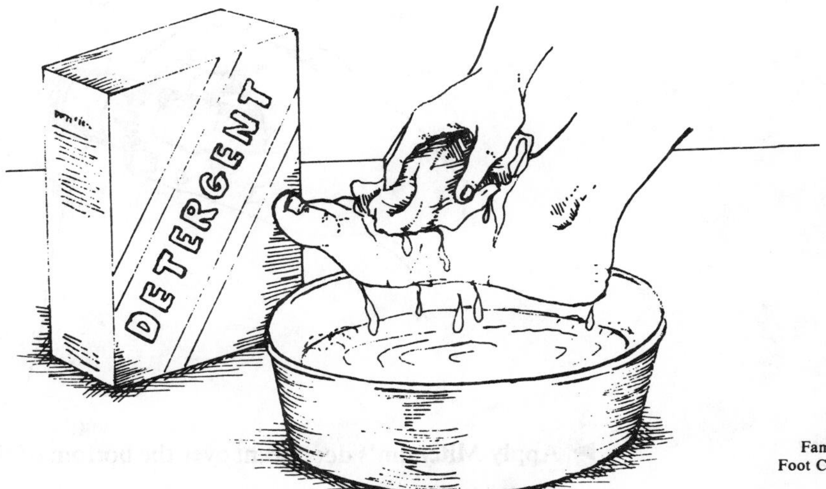

1. Thoroughly scrub the feet with a warm solution of laundry detergent. Use a wash cloth to wash and remove the dead skin.

2. Rinse feet thoroughly and dry with soft clean towel.

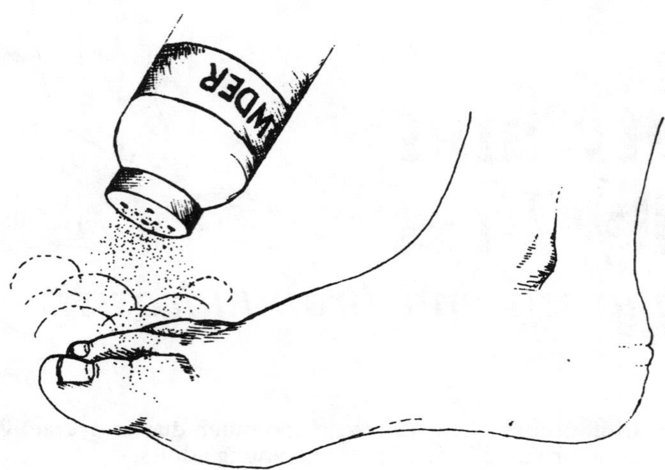

3. Powder feet liberally with medicated foot powder, and be sure to get it in between the toes. Tinactin powder and Aftate powder are two good commercial products for this.

4 If steps 1-3 don't do the job after a few days, try Mitchum's deodorant. Use it as follows:

► Wash foot thoroughly with rubbing alcohol.

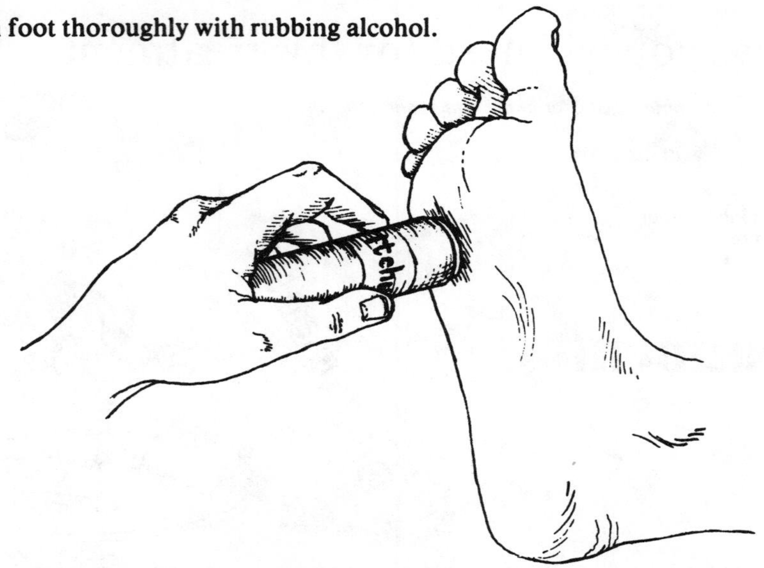

► Apply Mitchum's deodorant over the bottom of the foot at bedtime.

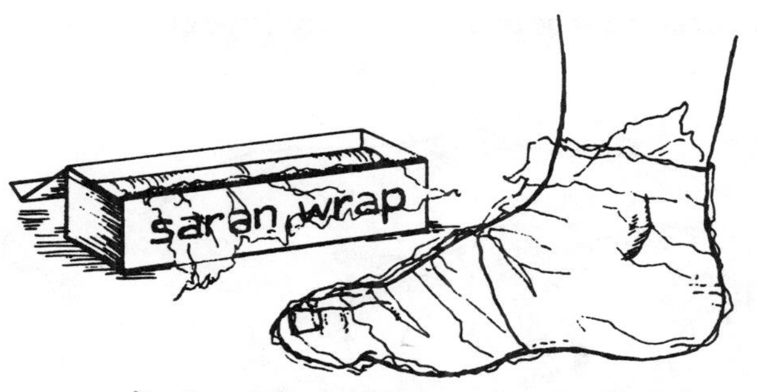

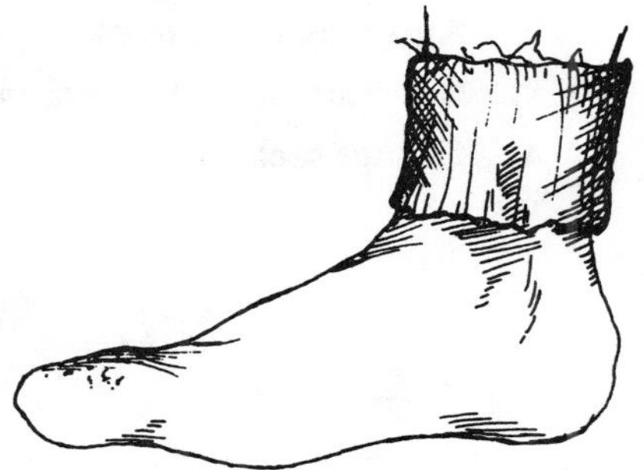

- Cover foot with saran wrap and sock.
- Wash off excess powder in the morning.
- Repeat process every night for one week, then once or twice a week as needed.

When to Call the Doctor

Sometimes excessive sweating and foot odor are caused by a mechanically unsound foot or an underlying fungus infection (Athlete's Foot). In these cases—or in any case where the treatment does not work within a few days—it is appropriate to consult a podiatrist.

DON'TS

- Don't wear the same shoes for two or more consecutive days.
- Don't wear shoes made of synthetics or leather substitutes which don't have pores and don't breathe well (see appendix on shoes).
- Don't use synthetic or nylon socks.
- Don't wear shoes without socks, especially in sports.

Practical Pointers for Prevention

1. Use the right kind of shoes for each of your activities.

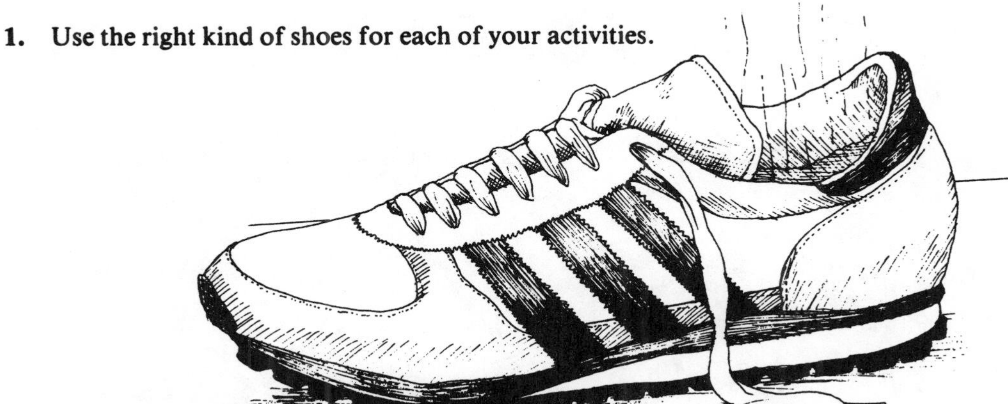

2. Air shoes out after use. It takes 24 hours for a shoe to dry out and reshape after using.
3. Use clean, absorbent cotton socks.
4. Change socks daily.

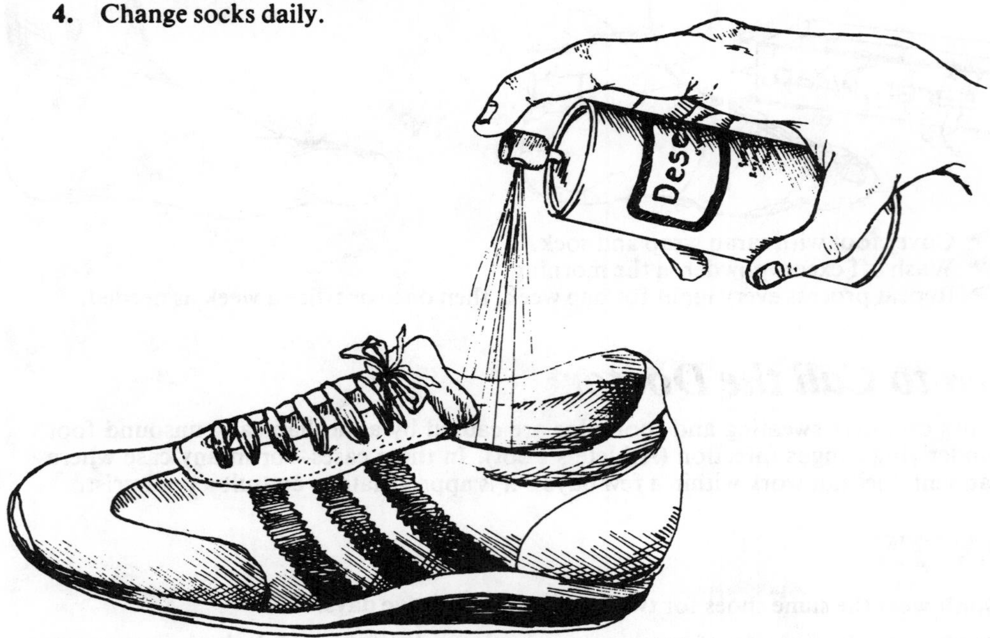

5. Spray shoes daily with Desenex or disinfectant before use.
6. Powder feet and socks liberally each day.

Chapter 14

Athlete's Foot

(Tinea Pedis)

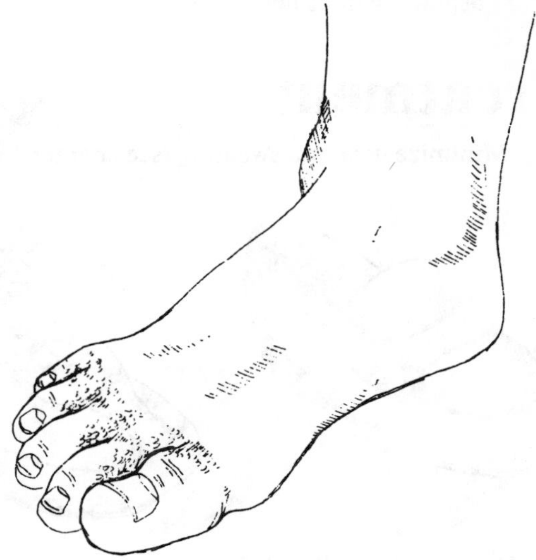

What is it?

Athlete's Foot (also called Ringworm) is a superficial fungal infection of the skin of the feet. It is a very common affliction, especially among males. In the early stages, fluid-filled blisters occur on the soles, sides or in-between the toes of the feet. Later, these areas become red, dry, scaly fissures. Dangerous secondary infections can occur if the primary (fungal) infection is not treated early.

Caution: ***Do not proceed with this treatment until you have read the Guidelines to Treatment in Chapter 2***

Things you will need for this treatment

see chapter 2 "Materials List" for brand names and substitutes

soap & water
antifungal liquid
medicated foot powder

Preparation for Treatment

► **Make sure any instruments you use are clean. Wash them in soap and water and rinse off with alcohol or some other recognized antiseptic.**

► **Make sure all materials and suggested medications are clean and up to date.**

► **Thoroughly scrub the entire foot with warm soapy water and a terry wash cloth. Pat dry with a soft clean towel.**

► Read through all the instructions which follow, and make sure you understand them before beginning treatment.

Treatment

1. Minimize heat and sweating (see chapter 13).

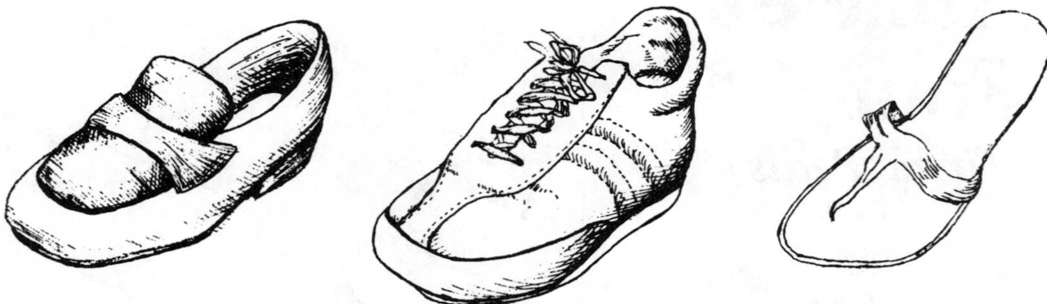

2. Wear well-ventilated shoes or sandals. Avoid using rubber or plastic shoes or boots (which prevent proper breathing).

3. Wear white cotton socks.

4. Apply Tinactin liquid twice during the day and once at bedtime.

5. Use an anti-fungal dusting powder such as Aftate or Desenex. Dust between the toes daily.

6. Continue treatment for two weeks after you think the condition has cleared.

CAUTION: If the area becomes red or swollen, or if it is draining, or isn't considerably improved within 2-3 weeks, see a podiatrist.

Practical Pointers for Prevention

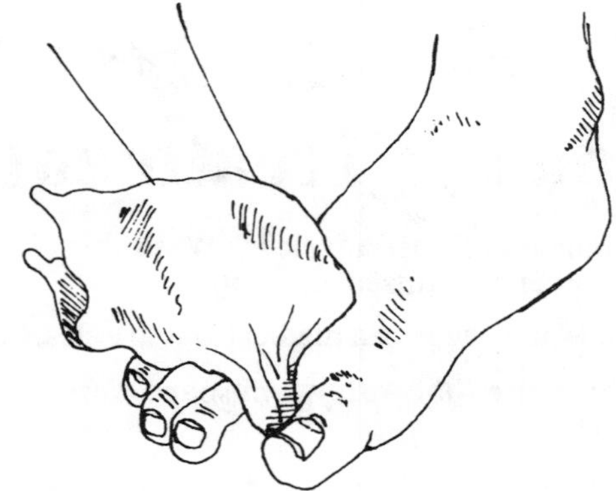

1. Wash the feet daily with mild soap and water, using a wash cloth or soft brush. Make sure you get between the toes.

2. After washing, dry thoroughly—especially between the toes.

3. If you are susceptible, use an anti-fungal powder daily and apply liberally between the toes and into the socks.

4. Wear cotton socks.

5. Avoid sweat socks and socks of synthetic materials, as they are good absorbers of heat—and therefore conducive to the environment in which fungi thrive.

6. Wear open-toed shoes or leather shoes of good quality that breathe properly. Be sure to change shoes and socks daily.

7. Always wear socks or stockings when wearing shoes.

8. Do not go barefooted.

9. When removing your shoes after a day's wear, air them out for 24 hours and spray them with an antiseptic spray such as Desenex before wearing again.

10. Avoid becoming overweight, as excessive weight leads to foot strain and excessive perspiration.

Chapter 15

Infection

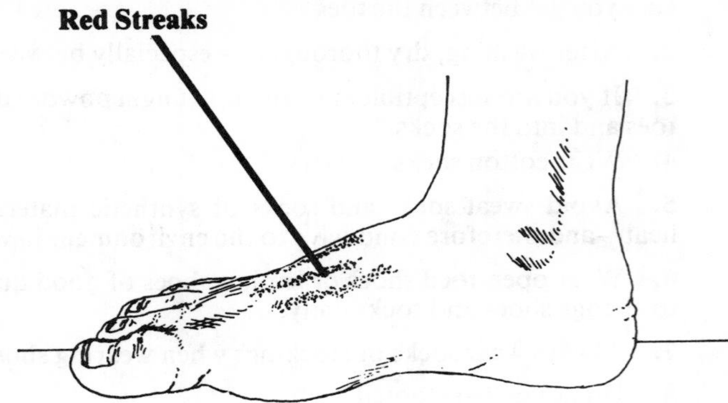

This chapter deals with infections of the skin, which are usually accompanied by redness, heat, swelling, pain and pus.

CAUTION: ***If you develop a temperature or notice red streaks or get chills, or if the symptoms of infection do not subside within 48 hours after you start treatment, see a podiatrist.*** Do not proceed with this treatment until you have read the Guidelines to Treatment in chapter 2.

Things you will need for this treatment

see chapter 2 "Materials List" for brand names and substitutes

soap & water
soaking solution
antiseptic
2"x2" gauze pads, sterile
antibiotic cream (if you have any)
adhesive tape

Preparation for Treatment

1. Make sure all the materials you will be using are clean and fresh as discussed in chapter 2.

2. Read through all the instructions which follow and make sure you understand them before beginning treatment.

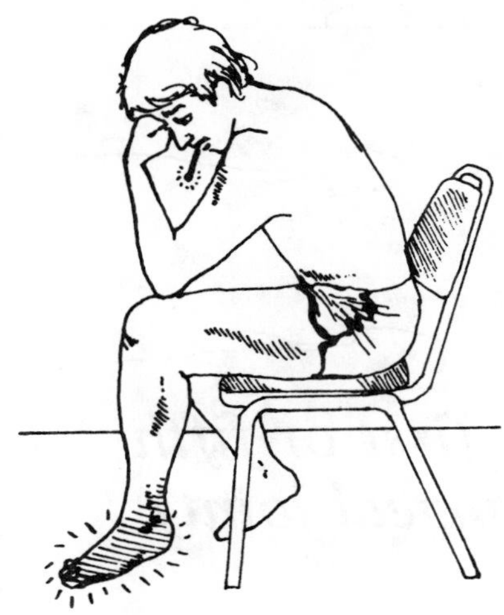

Treatment

1. Clean the area well with soap and warm water.
2. Soak for 20 minutes in warm water with Domeboro or epsom salts added, two to three times daily.
3. Rest and keep pressure off the area by padding around it when possible.
4. Put an antiseptic solution on the infected area after each soak, and then cover with antibiotic cream and 2x2 sterile gauze pads.
5. To control pain and/or fever, take two aspirin every four hours.

Chapter 16

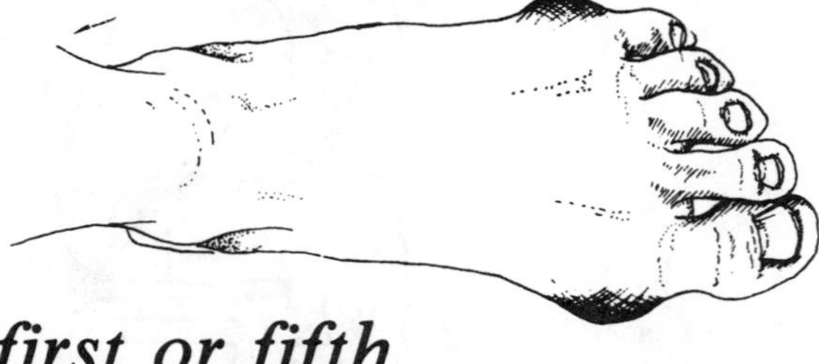

Bunions

(Bursitis of the first or fifth metatarsophalangeal joint)

What is it?

A bunion is an inflammation which can occur either on the outside of the big toe joint or the outside of the little toe joint. A "big toe" bunion is an enlargement of the outside of the head of the first metatarsal bone. The big toe may be straight, but is sometimes angled or pointed toward the small toe, subjecting the bony bump to a great deal of irritation. The skin and soft tissue around this bump become irritated and inflamed. The area may become red, hot, and swollen, and very painful. Continued pressure on this area can lead to the development of infection or the formation of corns over the bump. The small toe bunion, or Tailor's bunion, is an enlargement of the outside of the head of the fifth metatarsal bone. The little toe is sometimes pointed in toward the big toe, causing irritation to the enlargement. This area may also become red, hot, swollen, and very painful. Continued pressure on this area can also lead to the development of an ulcer, infection, or the formation of corns over the bump.

Things you will need for this treatment

see chapter 2 "Materials List" for brand names and substitutes
soap & water
adhesive spray and skin protectant
adhesive foam or felt 1/8" and 1/4"
2"x2" gauze pad
adhesive tape
moleskin or elastic adhesive bandage 3" square
heating pad
ice bag
aspirin
soft polyurethane foam 1/4"
cotton material 1" by 18"
nitrogen-impregnated foam innersole
bunion shield

Caution: ***Do not proceed with this treatment until you have read the Guidelines to Treatment in Chapter 2***

Preparation for Treatment

► Make sure any instruments you use are clean. Wash them in soap and water and rinse off with alcohol or some other recognized antiseptic.

► Make sure all materials and suggested medications are clean and up to date.

► Thoroughly scrub the entire foot with warm soapy water and a terry wash cloth. Pat dry with a soft clean towel.

► Read through all the instructions which follow, and make sure you understand them before beginning treatment.

Treatment

1. Apply tincture of benzoin to the irritated area.

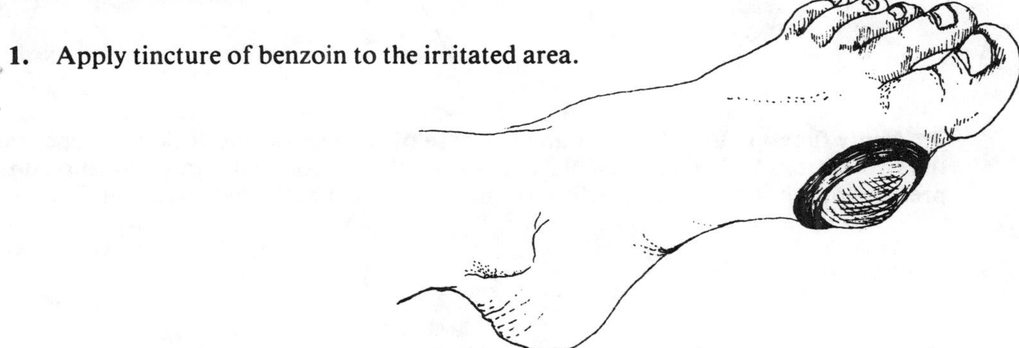

2. Remove the irritation from the bunion by padding around it with 1/8" adhesive felt. Cut a hole in the felt a little larger than the bump and trim the circumference of the pad so that there is 1/8" to 1/4" width of padding all around the bump. An alternative here is to use a commercially available "bunion shield."

3. Apply VASELINE™ into the hole, cover with gauze and tape down.

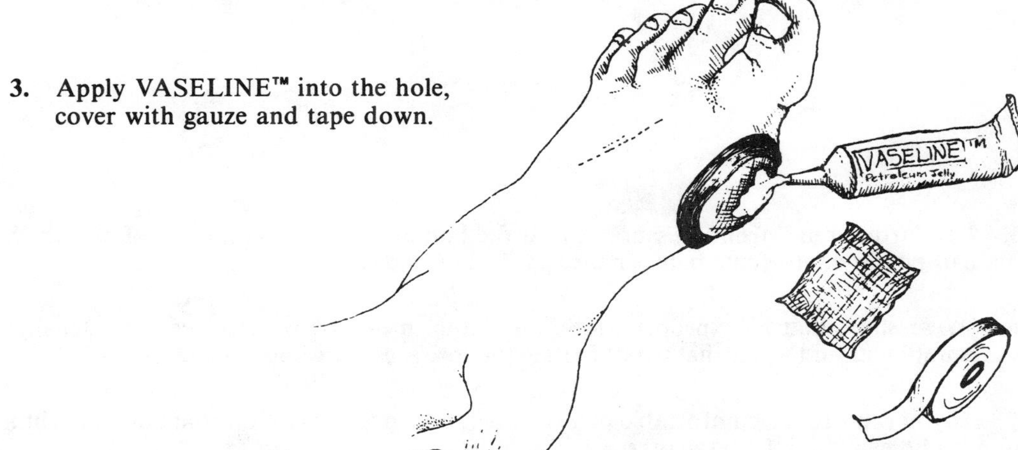

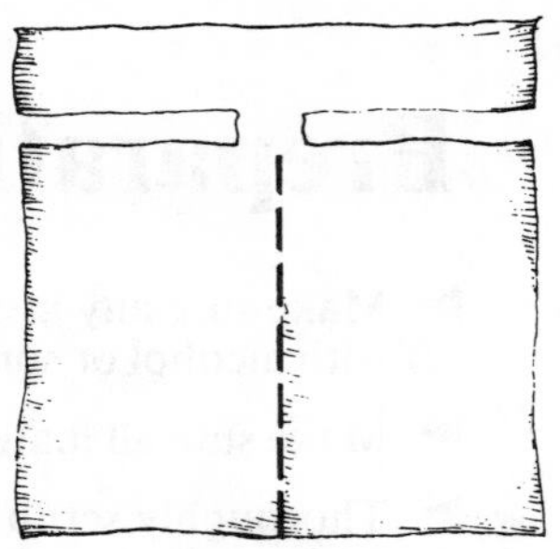

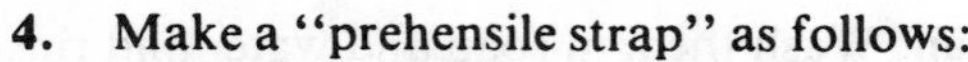

4. Make a "prehensile strap" as follows:

► Take a piece of 3"x 3" adhesive tape, Elastoplast©, or moleskin and fold it in half, sticky side up.

► Cut it into a "T" shape.

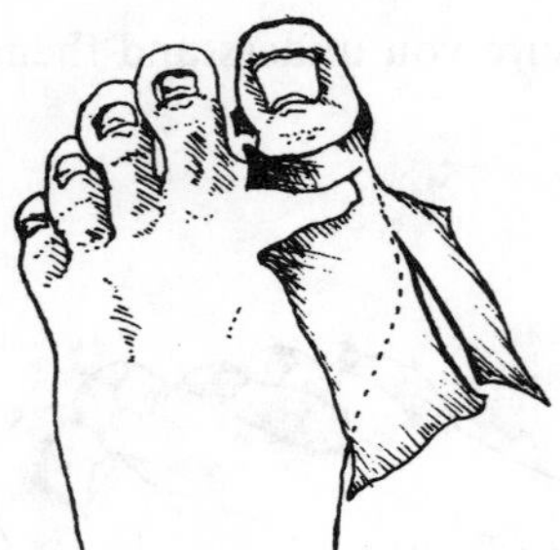

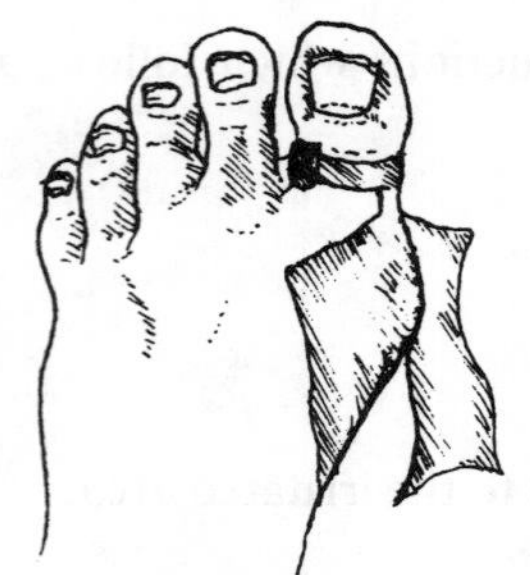

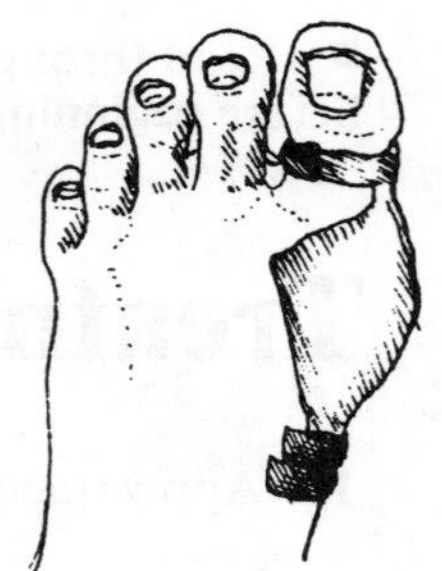

► Apply the top of the "T" around the base of the big toe and lock with tape. Pull the two bottom "T" flaps into place, covering the bunion. The strap will spread the pressure of the shoe against the foot so that it is not concentrated on the bunion.

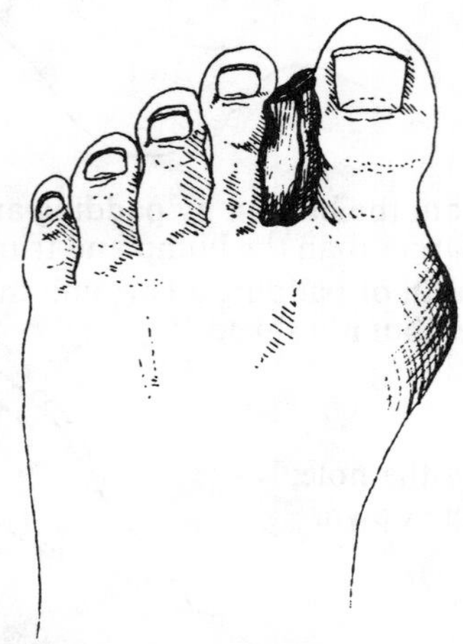

5. For further relief from pressure against the bunion joint, insert a piece of ¼" thick foam or polyurethane foam between the first and second toes.

6. Wear shoes that have proper width and depth in the toe box. If necessary, change shoes until you find a pair that won't irritate the sore area (see appendix on shoes).

7. If you can't find a comfortable pair of shoes, take one of the pairs you have and slit it or cut a hole in it to relieve the pressure.

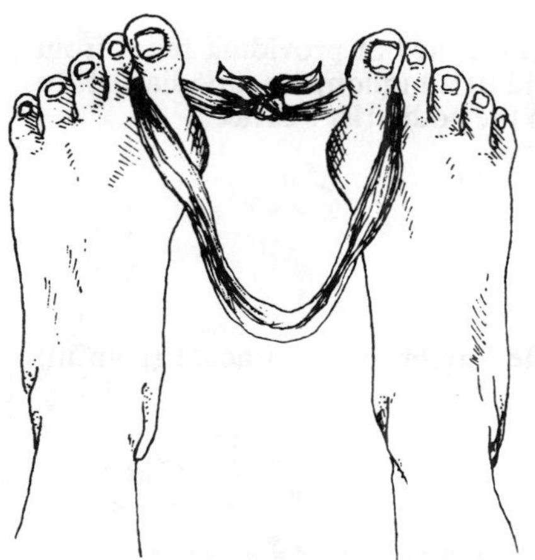

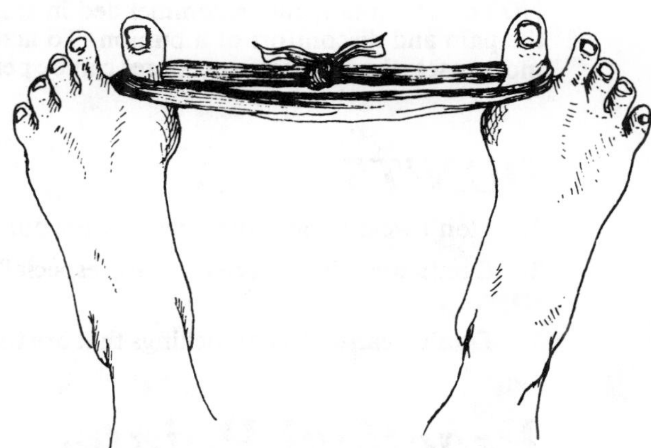

8. Make an exerciser that you can use every morning to loosen up the bunion joint and make it more mobile.

► Take a 1″ by 18″ piece of cotton material or thin rope.

► Tie a loop and place one end around each large toe.

► Keep heels on a flat surface, pull toes apart, and hold for five seconds. Start by doing this pull ten times a day, and increase one time each day until you get to 25 pulls a day.

9. After you have tried steps 1-8, if there is pain deep in the bunion joint, or if there is redness or swelling around it, try the following:

► Get off your feet (except for walking) for a few days.

► Use local applications of heat two or three times a day, with a heating pad, or with hot water soaks (see chapter 2).

► Take two aspirin every four hours for three days, then two every six hours for up to one week.

► When you resume normal activities, apply an ice pack for 15-30 minutes at the end of the day. If partaking in sporting activities or long walks, apply an ice pack for 15-30 minutes before and after the activity. Discontinue this step when pain is gone.

10. Once the acute stage is over, you may want to fit your shoes with a Spenco inlay.

► Make a varus wedge long enough to extend from the back of the heel to the arch (see appendix on making your own inserts).

► If you also have a callous present on the bottom of the ball of your foot, incorporate bi-plane padding made out of 1/8" foam onto the Spenco inlay (see chapter 8).

If you have a Tailor's Bunion . . .

If your bunion is on the side of the little toe, follow steps 1, 2, 3, 6, 7, 9, and 10 above. For step #2, the bunion pad, vaseline and 2x2 gauze can be all held down by a piece of moleskin cut out in an egg shape and anchored with two or three strips of "1" adhesive tape.

When to Call the Doctor

If severe swelling, redness, heat and pain persist for two days with no relief, or if you see a break in the skin and/or are running a fever, see a podiatrist.

NOTE: The treatments recommended in this chapter are aimed at providing relief from the pain and discomfort of a bunion. To actually get rid of a bunion, see a podiatrist. In most cases, the surgical procedures can be performed in the podiatrist's office.

DON'TS

1. Don't wear a shoe with a narrow toe box.

2. Don't wear high heeled shoes, especially when the bunion is in an acute (painful) stage.

3. Don't wear socks or stockings that are too tight.

Practical Pointers for Prevention

1. Make sure you wear properly fitted shoes, paying special attention to width and length. (See appendix on shoes).

- ► If you are an athlete, make sure you use athletic shoes with good toe box width and depth.
- ► If you are a runner, get running shoes with good forefoot shock absorption.
- ► Once the pain is under control, you may wish to purchase a commercially available "bunion shield" to wear daily.

Chapter 17

Pain in Front of Foot
(Morton's Neuroma)

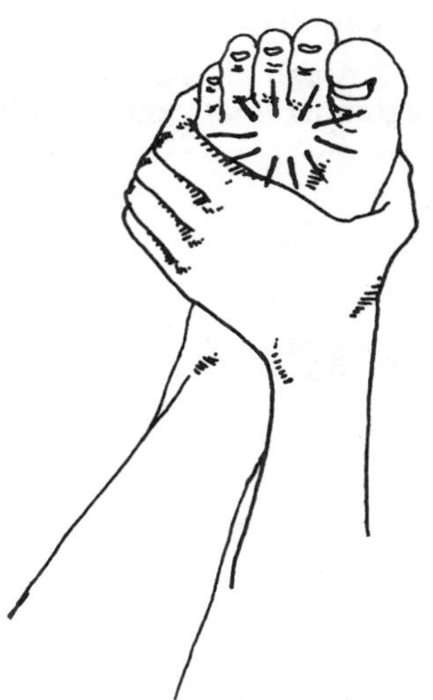

What is it?

Occasionally one of the small nerves in the front of the foot gets pinched between two metatarsal bones, causing tingling, numbness and/or pain extending from the adjacent toes into the front of the foot. This pain is especially noticeable if you squeeze the front part of the foot from side to side. This condition most commonly occurs between the third and fourth toes.

CAUTION: A painful burning sensation in the feet can be caused by many local (foot) as well as general (body) conditions. Local pain can be caused by poor circulation in the foot, athlete's foot (chapter 14), or a pinched nerve or neuritis such as Morton's neuroma (described above). However, a general burning sensation can also be caused by diabetes, anemia, thyroid disease, alcoholism, and other conditions. Therefore, if you do not get relief with what is suggested, see a podiatrist or a physician immediately.

Things you will need for this treatment

see chapter 2 "Materials List" for brand names and substitutes

wet heat
adhesive felt 1/8"
nitrogen-impregnated foam innersole
aspirin
ice bag

***Caution:* Do not proceed with this treatment until you have read the Guidelines to Treatment in Chapter 2**

Preparation for Treatment

1. Make sure that all the materials and medications you will be using are clean and fresh as discussed in chapter 2.

2. Read through all the instructions which follow, and make sure you understand them before beginning treatment.

Treatment

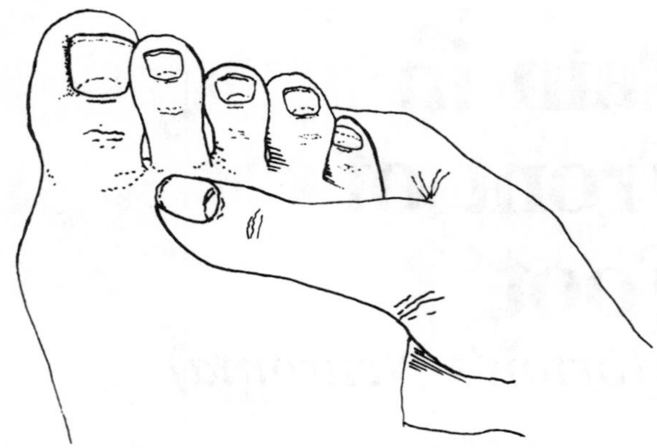

1. When the burning sensation occurs, remove the shoe and massage the toes and front of the foot. Move the toes gently up and down.

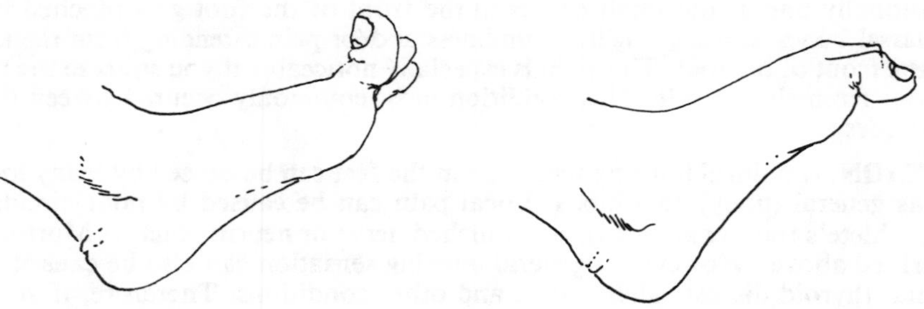

2. Do toe stretching exercises as illustrated.

3. Wrap a heating pad around the foot two times daily for twenty minutes each time on the medium setting. If you have a home whirlpool bath, use it with warm water.

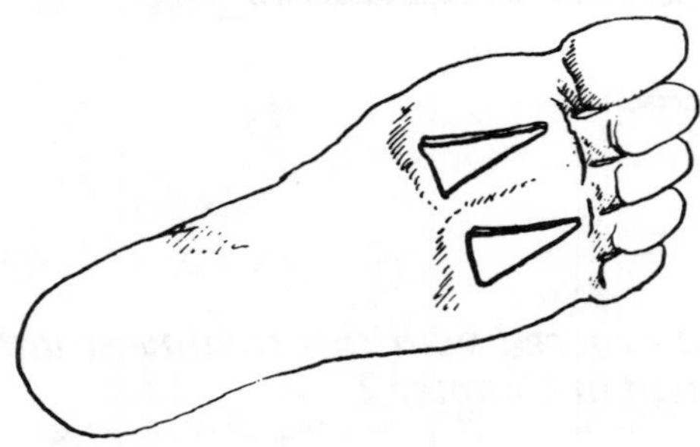

4. Place a triangular shaped pad cut out of 1/8" felt on the bottom of a Scholl or Spenco inlay to keep the bones which are irritated separated (see the section on callouses in chapter 8, and the appendix on Shoe Inserts You Can Make). You can also put this pad directly on the bottom of your foot.

5. Take two aspirin every four to six hours (for up to one week) to diminish inflammation and pain.

Practical Pointers for Prevention

1. Wear shoes that have these features:
   - ► A large toe box, giving the foot plenty of room in the front. (A narrow toe box will increase irritation.)
   - ► Low heels, to keep pressure off the ball of the foot.
   - ► Laces, buckles, or straps that permit adjustment of width.

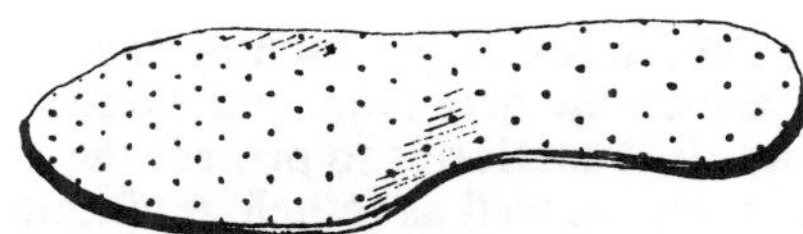

   - ► Thick, shock-absorbent soles. (For thin-soled shoes, you can try a Dr. Scholl's cushion sole or Spenco innersole—but make sure the insert doesn't cramp the toes. You may be able to stretch the shoe to accommodate the insert by filling a sock with sand, stuffing it into the toe box, and wrapping the shoe with a wet towel. Let it dry out over the next 24 hours. Repeat once or twice if needed.

2. If you are an athlete:
   - ► Add plain Spenco innersoles to running or athletic shoes to aid in forefoot shock absorption. Two pairs of Spencos, one on top of the other, will provide even more shock absorption.
   - ► Wear shoes with the widest possible toe box and the best possible forefoot shock absorption (see appendix on running shoes).
   - ► Ice the area down for 5-10 minutes after running, then apply heat later as previously discussed.

Chapter 18

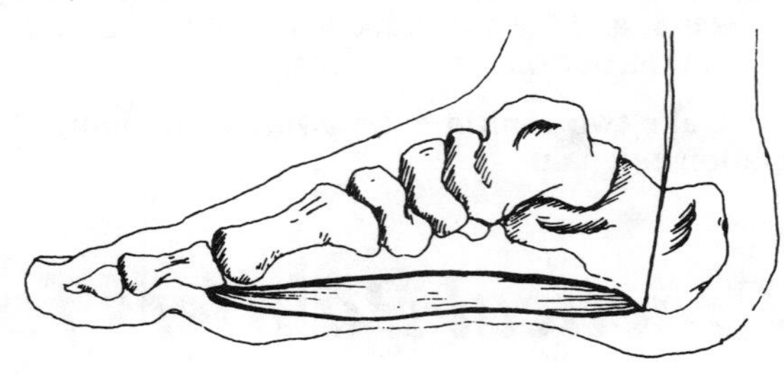

Arch Pain

(Plantar fasciitis)

What is it?

The strongest ligament in the body is the plantar fascia, a fibrous band of tissue that starts on the bottom surface of the heel bone and extends forward on the bottom of the foot to just behind the toes. Its function is to protect the softer muscles and tissues on the bottom of the foot from injury, as well as to help maintain the integrity of the foot structure itself. For pain along the outside arch on the bottom of the foot, the treatment is basically the same.

CAUTION: If the fascia becomes stretched or strained, or in some cases actually torn, the arch area becomes tender and swollen. This inflammation, called plantar fasciitis, is likely to be painful from the heel through the arch. In the early stages, there may be swelling and a feeling of rigidity (stiffness) in the arch.

Do not proceed in this treatment until you have read the Guidelines to Treatment in chapter 2.

Things you will need for this treatment

see chapter 2 "Materials List" for brand names and substitutes

soap & water
ice bag
foot roller
adhesive tape 1" and 1½"
adhesive spray and skin protectant
nitrogen impregnated foam innersole
adhesive felt ¼"
soft polyurethane foam
aspirin

Preparation for Treatment

1. Make sure all the materials and medications you will be using are clean and fresh as discussed in chapter 2.

2. Read through all the instructions which follow, and make sure you understand them before beginning treatment.

3. Thoroughly scrub the entire foot with warm soapy water and a terry wash cloth. Pat dry with a soft clean towel.

Treatment

1. Apply ice for intervals of 30 minutes (on for 30 minutes and off for 30 minutes) for as long as possible during the first 24-48 hours, to reduce the swelling and spasm.

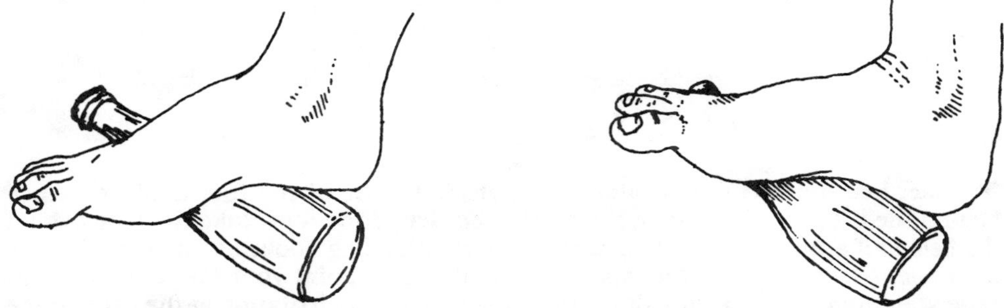

2. During the "off" periods, place a soda bottle on the floor, place your foot on top of it, and move the bottle back and forth from heel to toe. Do this for 2-5 minutes, three times daily, to help alleviate the swelling and spasm.

3. Rest, with very limited weight on the feet for 24-48 hours. After 48 hours, if you still feel pain, do not walk any more than necessary or participate in sports. When you are off your feet, elevate them.

4. Strap the foot as instructed below, to relieve pressure:

- ► Spray or paint tincture of Benzoin over the area of the foot to be taped.
- ► Cut three or four pieces of 1½" to 2" adhesive tape, each five to six inches long.

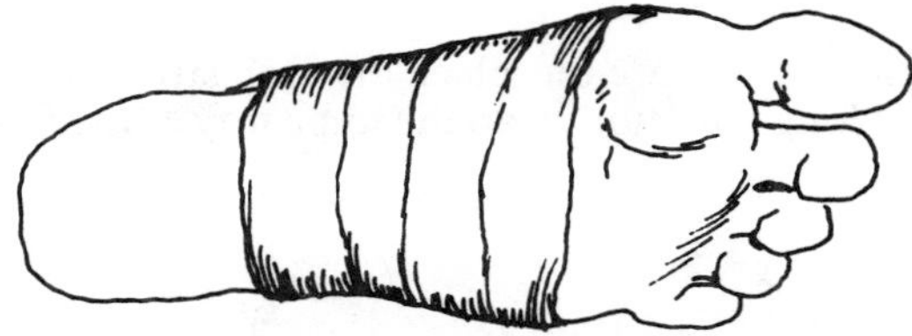

- ► Anchor each piece along the outside border of the foot and pull inward and upward with plenty of tension to support the arch. Start with the first piece of tape about one inch in front of the heel.

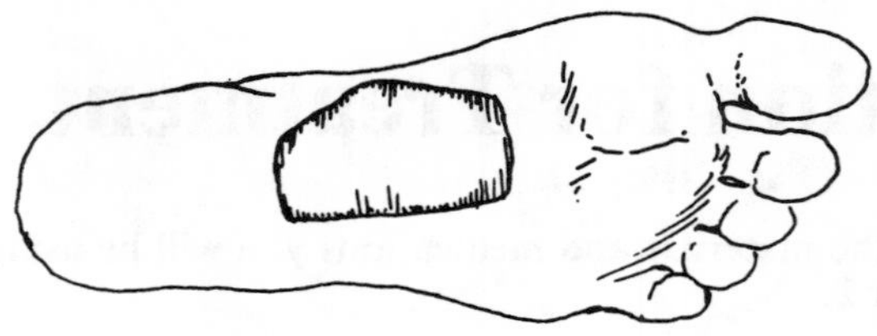

► If the tape alone does not seem to help enough, try using ¼" foam or felt padding cut to the contour of your arch as illustrated:

5. If this type of strapping does not provide enough support, carefully remove the tape (see chapter 2) and try using "retention" straps, as follows:

► Spray or paint tincture of benzoin over the area of the foot to be taped.

► Cut three strips of one inch tape approximately 8-12 inches long, depending upon your foot size.

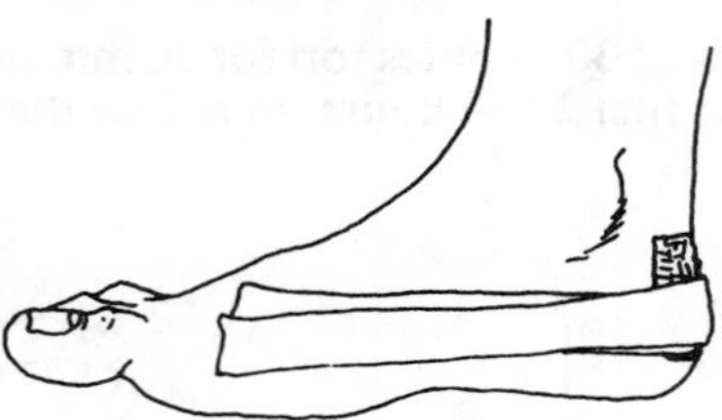

► Place one end of the tape along the outside border of the foot about one inch behind the little toe. Following the outside border of the foot, take the tape behind the heel and around to the other side of the foot, ending about one inch behind the large toe. (Before placing the tape down on the foot, point your toes downward to raise your arch up, then smooth the tape down. To avoid irritation at the back of the heel, before taping, place some vaseline over the heel and cover with a piece of gauze).

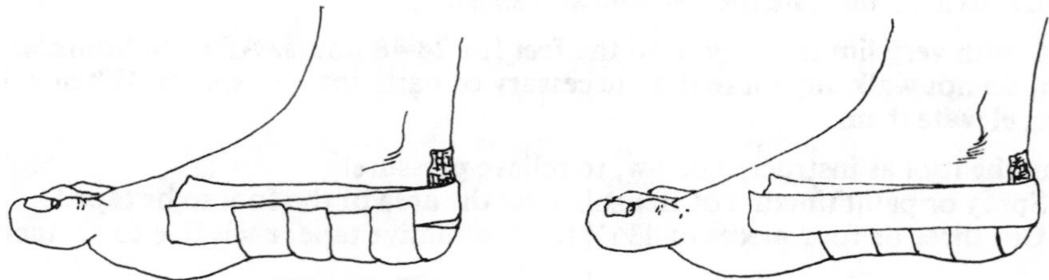

► After two retention straps are on, place the arch straps as described in step four. Then apply the third long retention strap the same way as the first two.

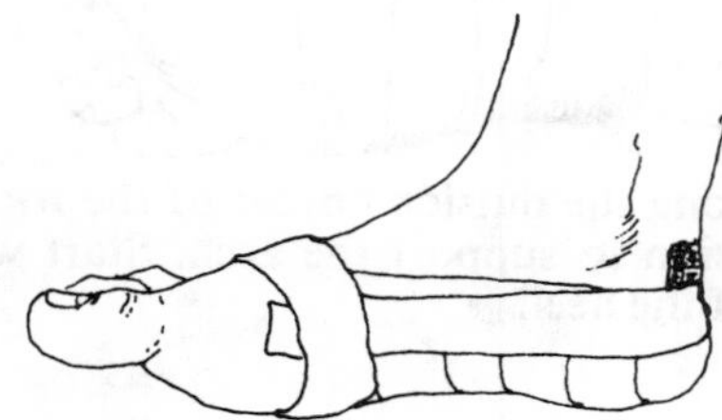

► All of this is finally anchored securely by placing one or two strips of 1½'' or 2'' wide adhesive tape on the top of the foot and ending underneath the arch on each side.

6. If pain is along the outer arch area, apply two retention straps and one "ankle eight" strap (run tape under arch and up around ankle and back under arch in "figure of 8" fashion). As long as pain and inflammation continue, take two aspirin every four hours (for up to seven days).

7. If you are an athlete, when returning to athletic workouts, apply ice before and after the workout for twenty minutes and again at bedtime, until all the pain is gone.

8. After the severe stage is over (this may take one to two months of strapping), keep the condition controlled by using a Spenco insole with an arch build-up attached to its underside, and if you pronate (roll in at the ankle) excessively, a ''varus wedge'' in the shoes. If you have a high arch, a ¼'' heel lift in each shoe may also be beneficial (see appendix on Shoe Inserts You Can Make).

9. Shoes with flexible soles should be worn for all activities, especially athletic workouts.

10. Excessive toe movement may aggravate this condition. To cut down on toe movement for at least the first six weeks after you've got this condition under control, try using an extra pair of socks or placing Spenco or polyurethane foam in the toe box of your shoes to make the toes fit more snugly.

When to Call the Doctor

If the pain and inflammation persist for more than five days after all of this treatment, or if you cannot bear weight on your foot, consult a sports medicine podiatrist.

DON'TS

► Don't go barefoot.

► Don't wear high-heeled shoes (over 1½ inch).

► Don't wear clogs, exercise sandals or negative-heeled shoes.

► Don't wear loafers.

► Don't run on the balls of your feet if you are prone to pain in the arch.

Practical Pointers for Prevention

1. Once the pain is gone and the problem is under control, use regular stretching exercises. Exercises which help to prevent recurrence include the wall push, push-ups on the toes, heels down on stairs, and rope pulls (see "Athletes' Health Care Book, From the Hip Down," Appendix on stretching.)

2. If you are a runner, avoid speedwork and hills until the condition is gone.

Chapter 19

Pain in Bottom of Heel

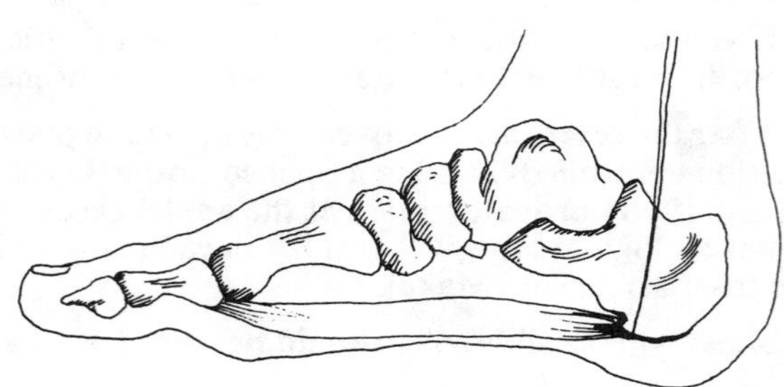

(Calcaneal spur, bursitis, or neuritis)

What is it?

Discomfort in the heel which is more than skin deep can have any of several causes.

- ► A *bone bruise* or *contusion* is an inflammation of the covering of the heel bone. It is painful in either walking or running.
- ► A *stone bruise* is a sharply painful injury caused by the direct impact of a hard object or surface against the foot (see chapter 21).
- ► *Plantar fasciitis* is an inflammation of the fibrous tissue band where it originates at the bottom of the heel bone. The pain often extends to the inside of the arch area and if you are a runner, is usually more severe when you are running faster or more on the ball of your foot (see chapter 18).
- ► *Nerve irritation* or *inflammation* is a condition which often afflicts the nerve just on either side of the heel bone extending down to the bottom of the heel.
- ► A *heel spur* is a shelf of bone, usually the entire width of the heel bone, formed by the continuous tearing away of the lining of the heelbone by the pull of the strong plantar fascia. Every time the lining tears, it heals forming a layer of new bone (calcium deposit) which eventually thickens to form 'The Bony Shelf.' This prominence digs into and irritates the surrounding tissue, usually giving rise to a *heel bursitis.*
- ► *Heel bursitis* is the formation of a protective sack of fluid, called a bursa, resulting from irritation caused by the spur. When this bursa becomes inflamed, it is called bursitis.

The latter two conditions, heel bursitis and heel spur, are often accompanied by pain and stiffness in the bottom of the heel, especially when you are getting out of bed in the morning. They often feel better after you have been walking on them for a few minutes. If you are a runner, you may also find that they are painful at the beginning of a run but start to feel better as the run progresses.

If swelling persists or recurs after a few days of rest, see a podiatrist. Similarly, if redness and heat are present, see a podiatrist. Remember, the problems covered here are the most common causes of pain in the bottom of the heel, but there are other possibilities—including conditions such as fractures, which should be treated by a podiatrist.

Caution: *Do not proceed with this treatment until you have read the Guidelines to Treatment in Chapter 2*

Things you will need for this treatment

see chapter 2 "Materials List" for brand names and substitutes

soap & water
antiseptic
ice bag
aspirin
a rope
adhesive felt or foam 1/8" and 1/4"
adhesive tape 1", 1½" or 2"
adhesive spray and skin protectant
nitrogen-impregnated foam innersole

Preparation for Treatment

1. Make sure all the materials and medications you will be using are clean and fresh as discussed in chapter 2.

2. Read through all the instructions which follow, and make sure you understand them before beginning treatment.

3. Thoroughly scrub the entire foot with warm soapy water and a terry wash cloth. Pat dry with a soft clean towel.

Treatment

The following treatment is designed for the heel spur syndrome, which can include at one time or another all of the different types of heel pain discussed above.

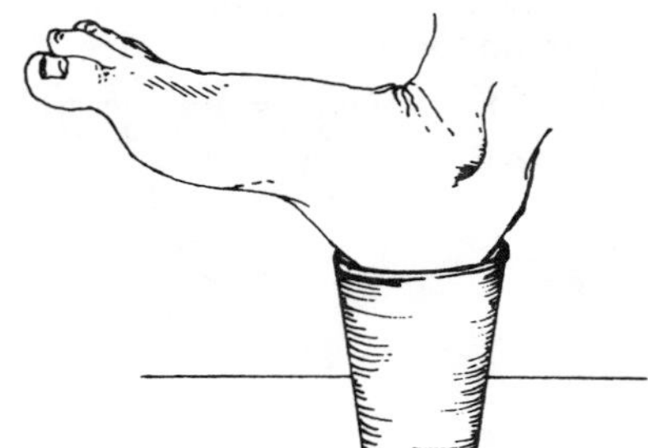

1. When you first have pain, apply ice to the bottom of the heel for 30 minutes.

2. Repeat the ice treatment at least two more times during the day, allowing 30 minutes for each application.

3. If swelling is present, elevate the leg (place the foot on two pillows above the level of the heart) as much as possible until the swelling diminishes. Plan on at least two days of rest from excessive standing, walking and/or running once the swelling has disappeared. If you swell up again when you try to run, double the amount of rest.

4. Use aspirin to help reduce inflammation. Take two aspirin every four hours for two to three days, then two aspirin every six hours for up to seven more days.

5. Pad the bottom of the heel to help take stress off the spot where the pain is. This padding can go directly inside the shoes. You can use heel cushion pads, sponge rubber heel pads, ¼" felt, or a piece of indoor/outdoor carpeting cut to the shape of the heel. Whenever you add a heel raise to an inlay or a shoe, you should do so for *both* feet, unless you are compensating for a leg length difference. The pad may be more comfortable if it is shaved down so the front part is a bit thinner (lower) than the back.

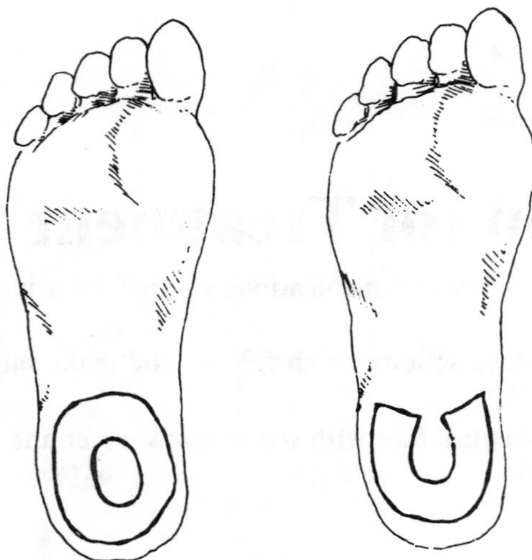

6. Note the specific spot where you feel pain, and cut a hole in the pad, making it a "donut." When in place, it will take direct pressure off the painful area. If there is discomfort because of the depression of the hole in the donut pad, then you can make it into a horse-shoe shape by cutting off the front part of the donut as shown.

7. If the problem is acute (occurred suddenly), it may be beneficial to tape the arches. Wash the feet first with soap and water and then clean them with rubbing alcohol. Apply tincture of Benzoin to all areas to be taped. Strap the area as instructed in chapter 18, steps 4 and 5.

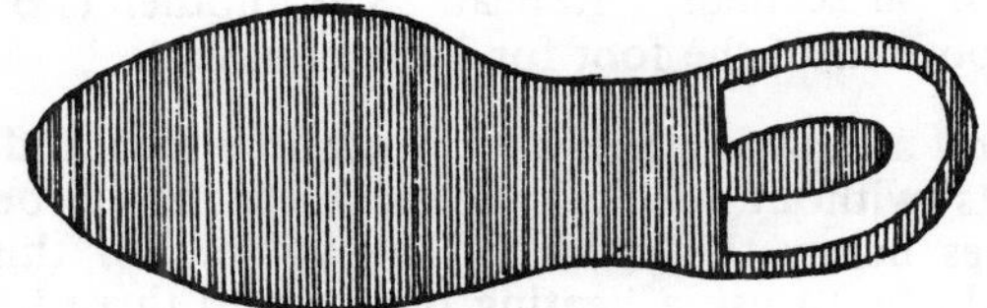

8. If the tape irritates your skin, purchase a pair of Spenco inlays. Put felt padding on the bottom surface of the Spenco inlays (chapter 18, #4), and from time to time, add to or replenish the felt build-ups as they wear down. You can also glue the heel pads you are using onto the bottom of the Spencos, so that they can easily be moved from one pair of shoes to another.

9. If you are bow-legged or have excessive shoe wear on the outside heels of your shoes, add a tilt of up to ¼" adhesive felt to the inside of the heel of your foot or to the Spenco inlay (see appendix on Shoe Inserts You Can Make). You can also put felt directly into the inside of your shoes, in the form of an arch pad, heel pad or "varus wedge" previously described.

10. If the pain is present on walking, keep the foot taped all day or wear the built-up Spenco inlays in all of your shoes. Other commercial insoles and inlays (such as Dr. Scholl's) are occasionally helpful, but making your own by applying felt build-ups onto the Spenco inlays is the most effective.

11. An additional aid to use with or without the various insoles discussed would be a plastic or rubber heel cup.

12. While convalescing, do not walk or run on your toes, as this will definitely irritate the condition. If you have a dull pain when you begin to walk or run but the pain goes away after a little while, you can continue to do so. If the pain gets worse as the walk or run goes on, stop!

13. Do the following series of stretching exercises daily. If they irritate the problem, they should be stopped or done with less intensity. As a rule, do the stretches slowly. Avoid bouncing or making jerky motions. If you feel burning in the back of the leg or bottom of the feet, you may be stretching too far and should ease off a little.

► Sit on the floor with your legs stretched out straight. Grasp your toes with your hands and pull slowly for 30 seconds. Repeat. Do another two 30-second stretches, using a rope behind the bottom of the foot for a better stretch.

14. If you think that you are having heel spur syndrome pain and have tried all of the recommended treatments without results, the problem could be an entrapment of cutaneous nerve branches below the inside of the ankle. For this condition, the appropriate treatment would be to use a heating pad two to three times daily for twenty minutes on medium heat and a varus wedge in your shoes (see appendix on Shoe Inserts You Can Make).

When to Call the Doctor

If you have followed all or most of these recommendations and are still having trouble with pain, redness, heat, or swelling, then see a podiatrist.

Practical Pointers for Prevention

1. Wear athletic shoes with good rearfoot shock absorption, a good heel counter for motion control, and good flexibility in the sole.

2. Make sure the shoes do not have excessive sole wear in the heel area.

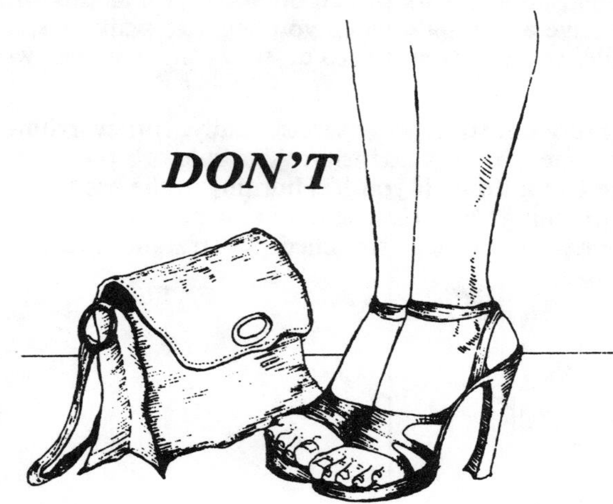

3. Don't use everyday shoes of more than 1½" in heel height; they can cause havoc with your feet. If you have a heel problem and are stretching the back of the legs in order to alleviate it, the use of built-up heels in your walking shoes will work against everything you are trying to accomplish with your stretching.

4. If you are overweight, lose weight.

Chapter 20

Back-of-Heel Pain

(Retrocalcaneal spur or Haglund's Deformity)

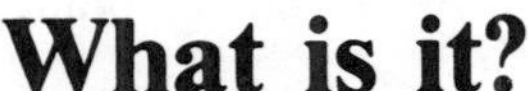

What is it?

A heel spur is a hard, usually painful area at the back of the heel where the achilles tendon attaches itself to the heel bone. When you squeeze this area you feel hard bone rather than the soft suppleness of the achilles tendon. Typically, the pain is not associated with any redness or blistering and is not brought on by squeezing the achilles tendon itself. The pain is usually located right below the achilles tendon where it attaches to the heel bone.

A Haglund's Deformity (pump bump) is an enlargement of the back of the heel bone. In many cases the pain in the heel is due to a bursitis which was in turn caused by the spur or Haglund's Deformity. The following treatment is applicable to all conditions associated with pain in the back of the heel, except blistering (chapter 21).

Things you will need for this treatment

see chapter 2 "Materials List" for brand names and substitutes

soap & water
ice bag
aspirin
rope
slant board
adhesive felt 1/8" to 1/4" or adhesive foam
nitrogen-impregnated foam innersoles
adhesive spray and skin protectant
heel cup

Preparation for Treatment

1. Make sure all the materials and medications you will be using are clean and fresh as discussed in chapter 2.

2. Read through all the instructions which follow, and make sure you understand them before beginning treatment.

3. Thoroughly scrub the entire foot with warm soapy water and a terry wash cloth. Pat dry with a soft clean towel.

Caution: ***Do not proceed with this treatment until you have read the Guidelines to Treatment in Chapter 2***

Treatment

1. Rest (keep off your feet as much as possible) for 24-48 hours. Use ice and elevation at least two or three times a day for 15 to 30 minutes each time.

2. Take two aspirin every four hours for two days, then every six hours for the next seven days (or until pain subsides).

3. After 48 hours begin ice therapy and the following exercises. Ice the back of the heel for six to twelve minutes or until the area is numb. Then do the exercises. Repeat the *ice*-exercise-*ice*-exercise-*ice* routine at least once and preferably two or three times daily, until there is no more pain. Take each stretch as far as you can—but if you reach the point where you feel a burning sensation, let up slightly and hold the stretch.

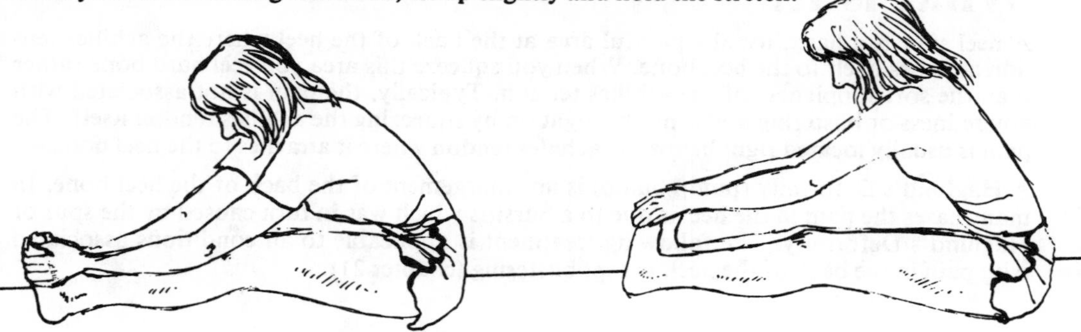

- ► Sitting down with the legs straight, grasp your toes and pull your feet slowly toward you. Hold for 30 seconds, then repeat.
- ► Do wall pushes with the back knee bent, then the back knee straight, two times each for 30 seconds. Only do this up to the point of pain.
- ► Do stair stretches for 30 seconds, twice.
- ► Do slant-board stretches for 30 seconds, twice.

4. Place heel raises in your shoes, starting with 1/8" and going as high as possible to try to take some of the stress off the back of the heel. A donut pad of foam rubber can be applied directly over the bump. See chapter 19, treatment #6.

5. If you are bow-legged or have excessive wear on the outside heel of your shoes, try placing a varus wedge on the inside of the heels of the shoes (see appendix on Shoe Inserts You Can Make).

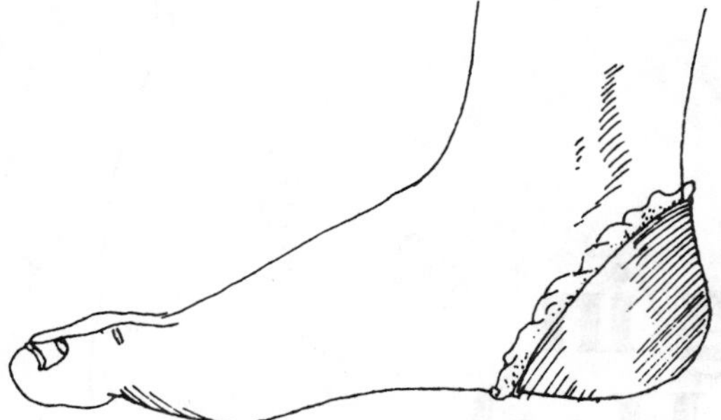

6. A plastic or rubber heel cup can be placed in the shoe to protect the spur or bump. It may be helpful to add a piece of 1/8'' foam to the inside of the heel cup.

7. If you feel any pain when you walk or participate in sporting activities, ice down for 15 minutes after exercising. Repeat later on that night. Once the pain is gone, discontinue icing.

8 Do not walk or run on your toes while convalescing, as this will definitely irritate the condition. If you are a toe runner, use a heel raise made of ¼'' felt thinned down in front.

9. If a dull pain occurs when you begin to walk or run, but disappears after a few minutes, you may continue. If the pain gets worse as you go on, stop!

When to Call the Doctor

If you have followed most of these recommendations and are still having trouble and there is pain, redness, or heat, then see a podiatrist. After four days, if the heel is swollen, see a podiatrist.

Chapter 21

Blistering in Back of Heel

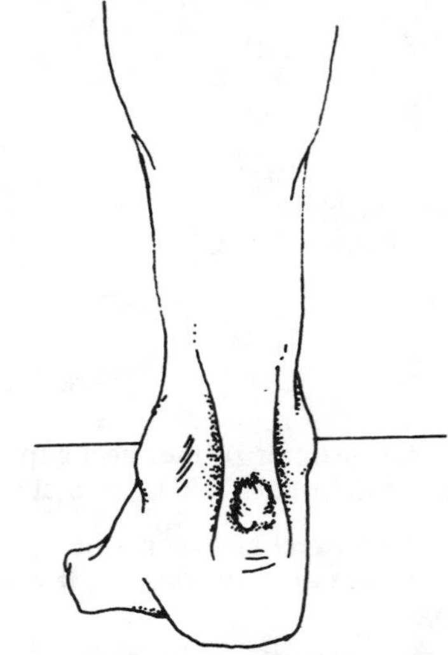

What is it?

Blistering in the back of the heel is a condition that can lead to painful retrocalcaneal bursitis and eventually to heel spurs on the back of the heel (chapter 20), if irritation is prolonged. It occurs when the skin at the back of the heel is caught between the pressures of the shoe counter (the back of the shoe) and the side-to-side motion of the heel bone. Immediate treatment may help to prevent progression to these more serious chronic conditions.

Things you will need for this treatment

see chapter 2 "Materials List" for brand names and substitutes
soap & water
ice bag
adhesive felt 1/8" and 1/4"
petroleum jelly
2"x2" gauze pads
adhesive tape 1½"
nitrogen-impregnated foam innersoles
adhesive spray and skin protectant
slant board
sole patching material
glue gun
rubber tips

Caution: *Do not proceed with this treatment until you have read the Guidelines to Treatment in Chapter 2*

Preparation for Treatment

1. Make sure all the materials and medications you will be using are clean and fresh as discussed in chapter 2.

2. Read through all the instructions which follow, and make sure you understand them before beginning treatment.

3. Thoroughly scrub the entire foot with warm soapy water and a terry wash cloth. Pat dry with a soft clean towel.

Treatment

1. Apply ice and compression to the back of the heel.

2. Take a steril pin (or the sterile tip of a scissors) and puncture the blister several times around its outer edges (see chapter 25).

To sterilize the pin or scissors' tip (a) place a lighted match to the tip, or (b) dip it into alcohol.

3. Squeeze the fluid out of the sides by applying gentle pressure to the top of the blister.

4. Leave the roof intact and clean with alcohol or soap and water, and pat dry with a soft clean towel.

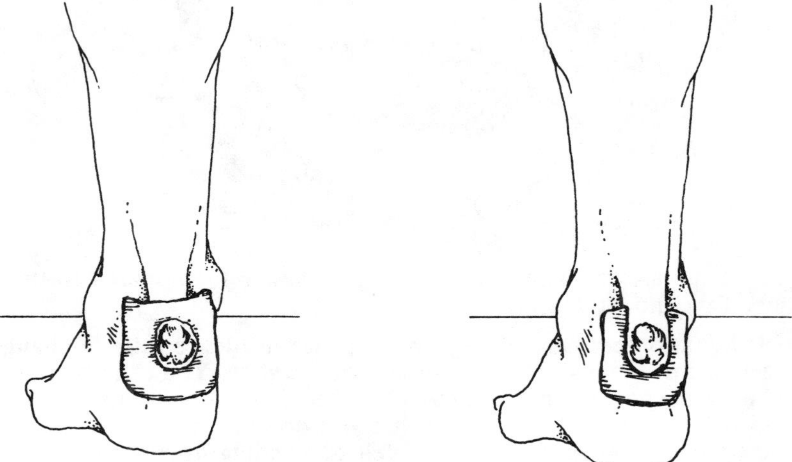

5. Cut a piece of 1/8'' felt into a donut or "U" shape a little larger than the blister.

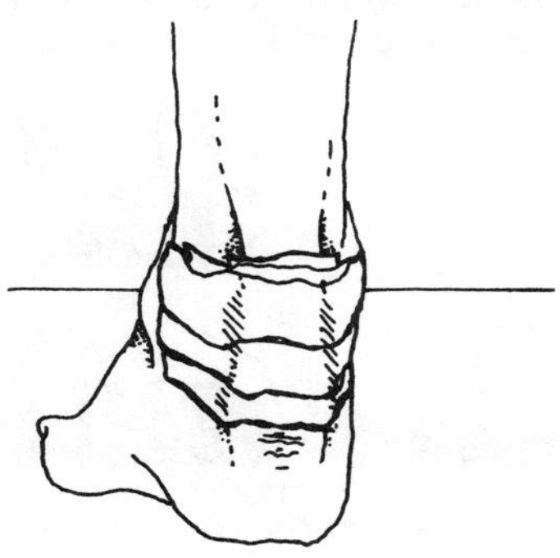

6. Lubricate the heel with VASELINE™ or A&D ointment. Cover with gauze and tape down. Leave in place (replace if necessary) for about a week.

7. Check to see if there is a seam on the inside part of the heel counter of the shoe that is causing this irritation to the back of the heel. If there is, cover it up with a piece of moleskin or tape, or get new shoes if necessary.

8. Repeat puncture and drainage procedure once a day if the fluid build-up recurs.

9. Sometimes heel blisters are caused by shoes which fit too loosely. If this is the case, add a layer of moleskin onto both sides of the back of the heel to make for a snugger fit. If the shoes are *very* loose, you can use ⅛" adhesive foam for this purpose, although it is preferable to purchase a new pair of shoes.

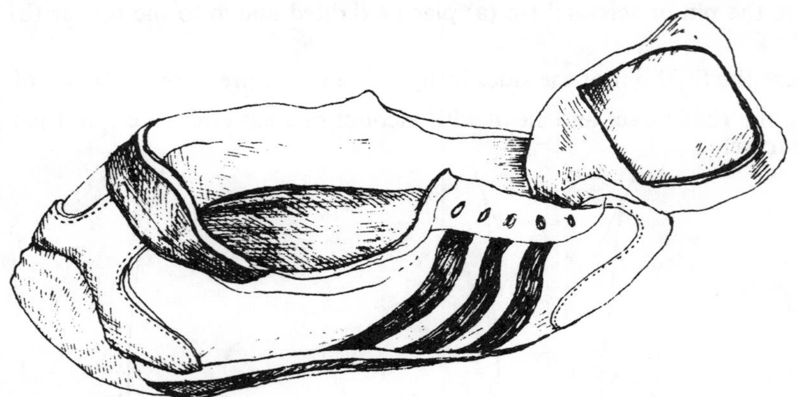

10. You can also try attaching 1/8" self-adhesive foam or felt to the underside of the tongue, if the shoe style allows.

11. If irritation persists, add a pair of Spenco insoles to raise or change the position of the heel against the inside of the counter of the shoe. You can use a heel raise to elevate and change the position of the back of the heel in relation to the heel counter. Make sure you do the same to both shoes, so that you do not cause an imbalance. The heel raise should be made out of 1/8" to ¼" felt (depending upon how high you need it), and placed directly in the shoe. It should be beveled down so that the front part is thinner.

12. As an alternative, glue the felt heel raise to the under portion of the Spenco inlay, so that the heel raise can be moved conveniently from one pair of shoes to another.

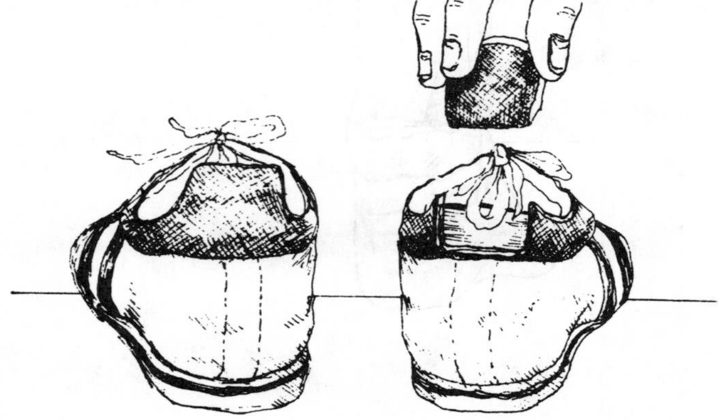

13. If the condition is severe, you can try cutting out the back of the shoe and sewing a piece of an ace bandage to the back of the shoe where you cut the counter out. Any elastic material will do if you do not have an ace bandage. A backless shoe also is helpful.

14. Try inserting a "varus wedge" in the heel of your shoe (see appendix on Shoe Inserts You Can Make). As an alternative, place this wedge on the bottom of a Spenco inlay instead of putting it directly in the shoe, so you can easily move it from one pair of shoes to another.

15. Do the following stretches each day before and after any extensive walking or athletic activity.

- ▶ Wall pushes with back knee straight, two times for 30 seconds each time.
- ▶ Wall pushes with back knee bent, two times for 30 seconds each time.
- ▶ Slantboard stretches, two times for 30 seconds each time.

16. Once you get the inflammation calmed down, 15 minutes of icing before and after extensive walking or athletic activity should help keep the problem under control. Discontinue icing once pain free.

When to Call the Doctor

If you think you have an infection (if the area is red, warm, or swollen), don't touch it yourself. See a podiatrist immediately.

Practical Pointers for Prevention

1. Make sure your athletic shoes do not have excessive sole wear in the heel area. If they do, you can repair them with shoe goo or shoe patch, or have the shoe resoled or replaced.

2. Make sure your shoes are properly fitted. If they are too loose in the heels, build up the insides of the shoes as described in Treatment sections #9 and #10.

Chapter 22

Stone Bruises

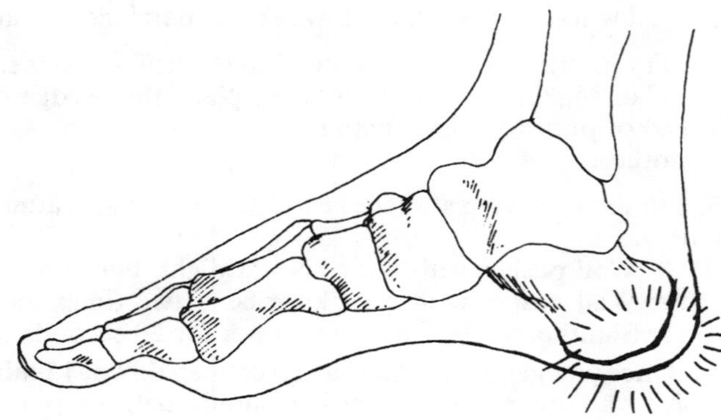

What is it?

A stone bruise is a sharply painful injury caused by direct impact of a hard object or surface against the foot. A stone bruise can be differentiated from other bottom-of-heel pain problems (see chapter 19) in that it occurs suddenly rather than gradually.

Things you will need for this treatment

see chapter 2 "Materials List" for brand names and substitutes

soap & water
antiseptic
ice bag
aspirin
adhesive felt or foam 1/8" and 1/4"
adhesive tape 1", 1½" or 2"
adhesive spray and skin protectant

Preparation for Treatment

► **Make sure all materials and suggested medications are clean and up to date.**

► **Thoroughly scrub the entire foot with warm soapy water and a terry wash cloth. Pat dry with a soft clean towel.**

► **Read through all the instructions which follow, and make sure you understand them before beginning treatment.**

Caution: *Do not proceed with this treatment until you have read the Guidelines to Treatment in Chapter 2*

Treatment

1. When you first have pain, apply ice to the bottom of the heel for 30 minutes.

2. Repeat the ice treatment at least two more times during the day, allowing 30 minutes for each application.

3. If swelling is present, elevate the leg (place the foot on two pillows above the level of the heart) as much as possible until the swelling diminishes. Plan on at least two days of rest from excessive standing, walking, and running once the swelling has disappeared. If you swell up again when you try to run, double the amount of rest.

4. Take two aspirin every four hours for two to seven days, depending on how long the pain continues.

5. Spray tincture of benzoin on the bottom of and back of the heel.

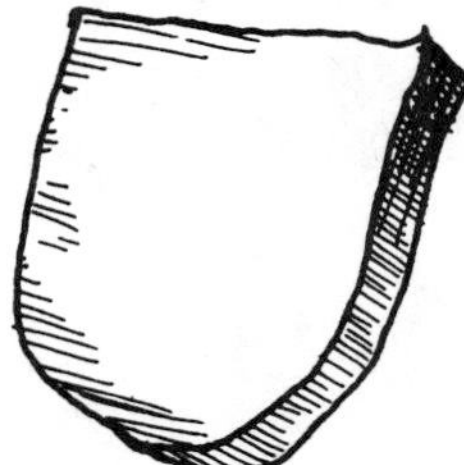

6. Cut 1/8" adhesive foam to the shape of your heel. Place the pad on your heel.

7. Apply four 6" strips of 1½"-2" adhesive tape to the pad, as follows:

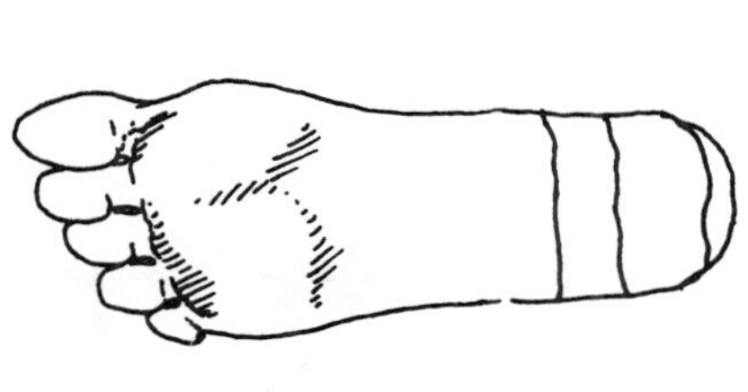

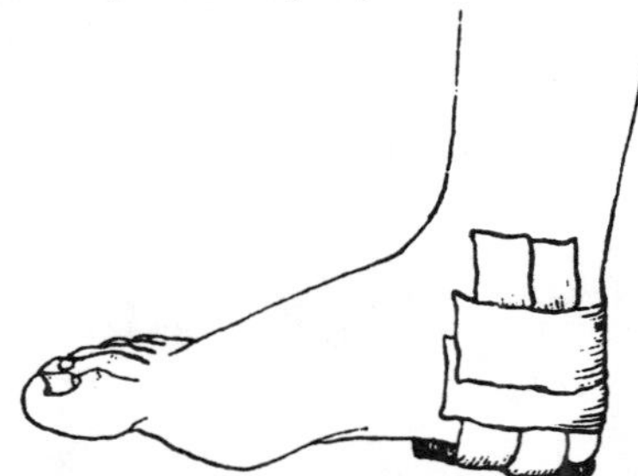

► Center one strip on the bottom of the heel pad and pull upward on both sides, attaching to the sides of the heel.
► Repeat with the second strip slightly behind the first, so that the bottom of the heel pad is covered.
► Center the third strip on the *back* of the heel (starting about one inch up from the bottom of the heel), pull around the heel and attach on the sides.
► Place the fourth strip so that it overlaps the third.

8. As an alternative (or an addition) to #7, place a properly fitted Spenco inlay in your shoes. If you wish, attach the cushion described in #6 to the bottom of the Spenco so that it can be moved easily from one shoe to another.

9. Additional relief can be obtained by using a heel cup padded with moleskin or 1/8" foam (see illustration in chapter 20, treatment #6).

10-13. Follow treatment steps 7-10 in chapter 19.

When to Call the Doctor

If you have followed all of the recommendations above, and the pain and swelling persist, then seek professional evaluation from a podiatrist to determine whether you have sustained a stress fracture or any other condition requiring a doctor's attention.

Practical Pointers for Prevention

1. Make sure your shoes do not have excessive sole wear, especially in the heel. If they do, have the soles repaired or replaced.

2. When resuming athletic activity, make sure you have shoes with good rearfoot shock absorption and a flexible sole.

Chapter 23

Cuts and Bruises

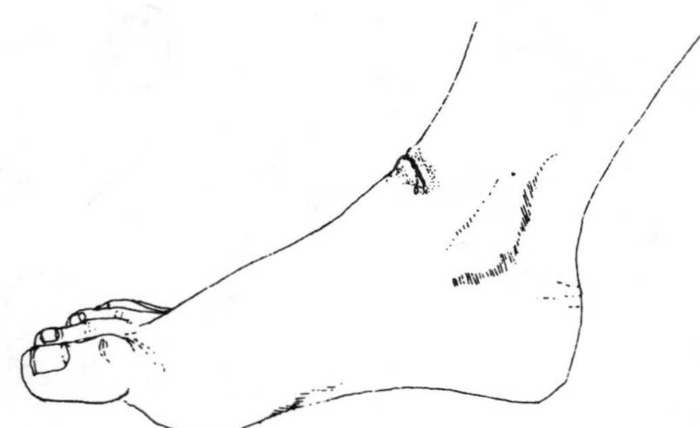

If a cut or bruised area is bleeding, but the bleeding can be controlled within a short period of time, it is likely that stitches are not necessary and that the injury can be treated at home.

Things you will need for this treatment

see chapter 2 "Materials List" for brand names and substitutes

soap & water
2"x2" gauze pad sterile
ice bag
ace bandage
pillows, 2
bandaids ("butterfly")

Preparation for Treatment

1. Make sure all the materials and medications you will be using are clean and fresh as discussed in chapter 2.

2. Read through all the instructions which follow, and make sure you understand them before beginning treatment.

3. Thoroughly scrub the entire foot with warm soapy water and a terry wash cloth. Pat dry with a soft clean towel.

Caution: *Do not proceed with this treatment until you have read the Guidelines to Treatment in Chapter 2*

Treatment

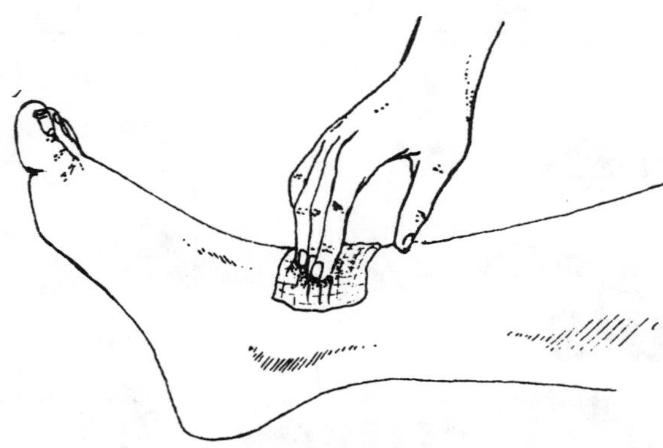

1. Cover the wound with a 2"x 2" sterile gauze pad and apply direct pressure on it for fifteen minutes. If the bleeding does not stop, re-apply pressure for another fifteen minutes.

2. Once the bleeding subsides, place an ice pack around the area for another fifteen minutes.

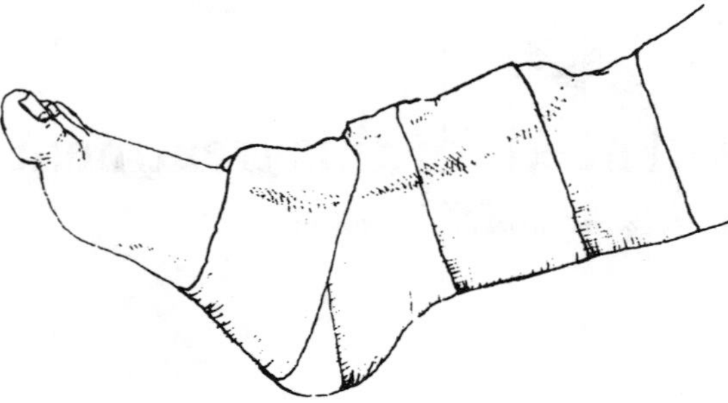

3. Cover the ice pack with an ace bandage and wrap around the area for compression. If mild bleeding continues, keep the foot elevated above the level of the heart (on two pillows) for several hours.

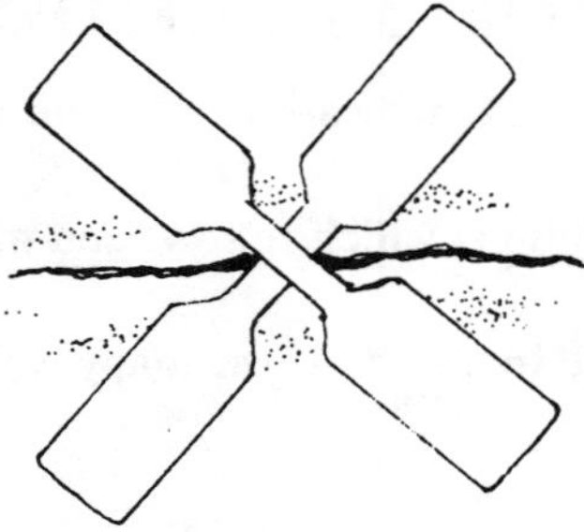

4. Once the problem is under control, apply bandaids in a criss-cross fashion to bring the wound edges together. So-called ''Butterfly'' bandages are specifically designed for this purpose and can be purchased at the drug store.

5. Ice can now be applied for the next 48 hours if necessary. Inspection of the area during the first couple of days may show some heat and swelling present, but this does not necessarily mean infection. It usually takes from 48 to 72 hours for an infection to occur.

When to Call the Doctor

If after two or three days the pain increases, the area feels hotter, and you see some oozing or pus, then you probably do have an infection. Another symptom of infection would be an increase in body temperature. If you think you have an infection, refer to chapter 15 or see a podiatrist. Don't use a tourniquet for a cut. It will only complicate the problem.

If the Injury Is a Puncture...

A puncture is a relatively deep hole in the flesh caused by a penetrating instrument such as a nail or knife. It usually bleeds less than an open cut, because the break in the skin is narrower. Use the same treatment for a puncture as you would for an open cut (above), but let it bleed for five to ten minutes because the wound is likely to be deeper and therefore more difficult to clean out. Make sure that you are especially careful in cleaning the area with soap and water.

If there is any dirt on the object which caused the puncture, you might need a tetanus shot and should see a podiatrist or a physician. Usually a tetanus booster is needed once every five years.

DON'TS

► Don't walk barefoot in city streets, alleys, empty lots, or other places where glass, nails, and trash are commonly found.

► Don't use a tourniquet for a cut. It will only complicate the problem.

Chapter 24

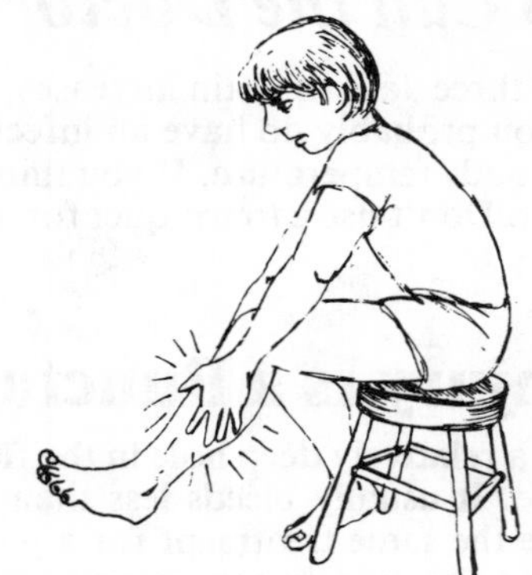

Cramps

"Growing Pains" in Children

A muscle working at a mechanical disadvantage because of *faulty body mechanics,* whether in the back, foot, or elsewhere, is subject to abnormal fatigue. If the disadvantage is large enough, the muscle will become weaker rather than stronger.

Muscle cramps and "growing pains" may be caused by chronic muscle strain and fatigue. They commonly occur in the calves and in the muscles of the feet. They are most often associated with flat (pronated) feet and with foot strain caused by "tight heel cords" in which there is a continuous contraction of the calf muscle. Tight muscles in the back of the legs and thighs, including contracted hamstrings, are often present. Muscle cramps are probably initiated by over-use and over-stress, resulting in a lack of oxygen delivery to the tissues.

Treatment should be aimed at correcting the mechanical abnormality. For example, when cramps are caused by foot strain, the child's feet should be given more support under the arch, and the contracted calf and hamstring muscles should be stretched.

Things you will need for this treatment

see chapter 2 "Materials List" for brand names and substitutes

nitrogen-impregnated foam innersoles
non-adhesive felt ¼"
slant board
weights 2 pounds and 5 pounds
aspirin
baby oil
adhesive felt 1/8"
wet heat

Caution:* *Do not proceed with this treatment until you have read the Guidelines to Treatment in Chapter 2

Preparation for Treatment

► Make sure all materials and suggested medications are clean and up to date.

► Read through all the instructions which follow, and make sure you understand them before beginning treatment.

Treatment

1. Fit a pair of Spenco inlays into the child's shoes.

2. Make a varus wedge, long enough to extend from the back of the heel to the arch (see appendix on Shoe Inserts You Can Make). Fix the inserts to the Spencos, so they can be moved from shoe to shoe.

3. Have the child do the following exercises four times a week. For each exercise, each leg should be stretched for 30 seconds twice.

► Wall pushes with the back leg straight
► Wall pushes with the back leg bent inward
► Hamstring stretches
► Toe touches
► Slantboard stretches

If your child is unable to do these exercises unassisted, then do the following.

► Have the child lie on his or her back, with legs extended straight. Grasp one of the child's feet, near the toes, and push it toward the knee for 30 seconds (if the child complains of pain, ease off until there is no pain). Release and then repeat.

► Repeat the above with the leg slightly bent at the knees, for 30 seconds, twice.

► With the child in the same position (flat on back) with one leg locked at the knee (straight), grasp the bottom of the foot and the back of the ankle and raise the entire straight leg up as far as possible (if the child complains of pain, pull back slightly). Hold this position for one or two seconds and slowly lower the leg. Repeat 20 times for each leg.

► Have the child sit on a table with legs hanging down. Hang two pounds of weight from the top of his foot (use an old pocketbook with a strap, or a paint can with a padded handle, and fill with rocks or other objects to the desired weight). Have the child pull his toes toward his face, without moving his leg. Repeat five times, holding for five seconds each time. Then do the same exercise with the foot turned inward.

Do all of the exercises above twice a day, four days per week.

4. Give aspirin (under age 12 use children's dose), two at bed time and two more as needed every 4-6 hours.

5. If the child walks on his toes or bounces conspicuously, make a heel raise of ¼" felt, and thin down toward the front (see appendix on Shoe Inserts You Can Make).

DON'T

► Don't allow the child to walk barefooted.

► Don't allow the child to wear negative-heel shoes (shoes in which the heel is lower than the forefoot).

When to Call the Doctor

"Growing pains" should never be written off as something that will automatically go away as the child gets older. They are symptoms of problems that can be corrected at an early age but become irreversible in adulthood. If home treatment does not bring relief from this problem after one or two weeks, see a podiatrist.

Night Cramps in Adults

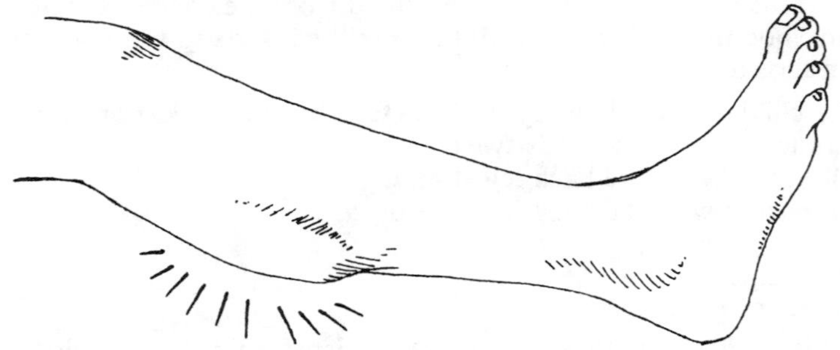

The cramps which occur in the muscles of the feet or legs at night—the so-called night cramps—are not symptoms of circulatory disorders of any kind. (Cramps occurring from poor circulation occur only as a result of exercise, and promptly disappear after a period of rest). Night cramps occur only during rest, and most often in bed. These muscle cramps are usually brought on by a sudden, exaggerated stretching of a muscle against little or no resistance from other muscles. They most commonly occur in the calf muscles (the strong muscle group in the back of the lower leg), but can also occur in the arch and toes.

Treatment

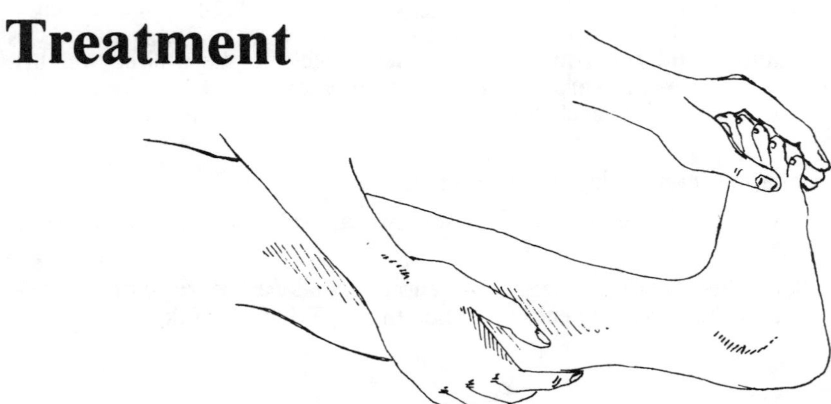

1. Immediate relief can be obtained by grasping the cramped limb with the hands and slowly but firmly helping it move in the opposite direction from the way the cramps have made it move.

► For calf muscle cramping (when the calf muscle knots up), grasp the foot with one hand and the calf with the other and slowly pull the foot upward (toward the leg). Hold this position until the calf muscle knot is released.

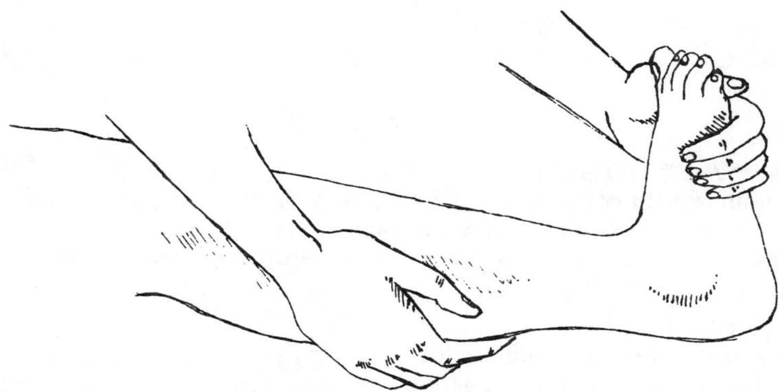

► For arch or toe cramping, hold the arch with one hand and toes with the other, and slowly pull the toes and the foot toward your face. Hold this position until the cramping sensation disappears.

2. Take some baby oil, apply liberally to the cramped area and gently massage the calf, arch, and/or toes for five to ten minutes with a back and forth motion.

3. Take two aspirin immediately and two more after four hours.

4. For longer term relief, fit a pair of Spenco inlays into your shoes.

5. Make a varus wedge long enough to extend from the back of the heel to the arch (see appendix on Shoe Inserts You Can Make). Attach to bottom of Spenco inlays in proper position:

   ► For calf cramps, add a heel pad made of 1/8″ felt and place on top of the varus wedging on the bottom of the Spenco inlay. This heel pad is made by cutting 1/8″ felt into the shape of the heel, and attaching it to the bottom of the varus wedge at the heel.

6. Apply moist heat applications to the affected muscle three times a day until there is no trace of cramping (see chapter 2).

7. Do the following exercises four to seven days a week. For each exercise, each leg should be stretched for 30 seconds twice.

   ► Wall pushes with the back leg straight
   ► Wall pushes with the back leg knee bent inward.
   ► Hamstring stretches
   ► Toe Touches

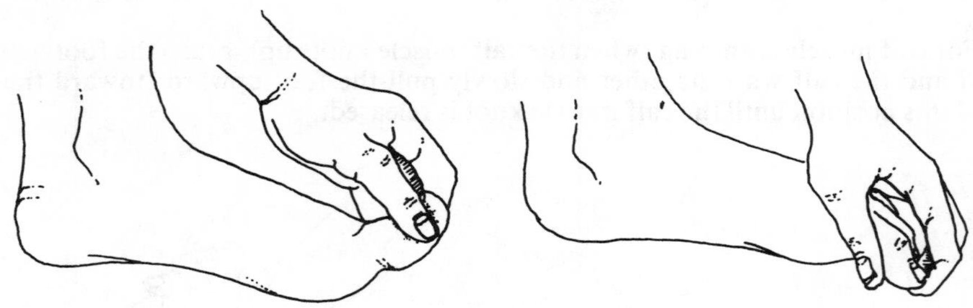

For Arch and/or Toe Cramps Only:

► With your weight off your feet (sitting or lying on your back), move your toes up and down as far as possible ten times in each direction.

► From a flat-footed standing position, move up and down on your toes 10 to 20 times.

For Calf Cramps Only:

► Sit on a table with legs hanging down. Hang five pounds of weight from the top of your foot (use an old pocketbook with a strap or a paint can with a padded handle, and fill with rocks or other objects to the desired weight).

► Pull your forefoot toward your face, without moving your leg. Repeat five times, holding for five seconds each time.

► Repeat the same exercise with the foot turned inward.

► Do these exercises twice a day, four days per week.

DON'T

► Don't walk barefooted.

► Don't use negative-heel shoes (shoes in which the heel is lower than the forefoot).

When to Call the Doctor

If after following the above recommendations, no relief is obtained within one or two weeks, see a podiatrist. If heat or swelling are present and/or if you have a fever, see a podiatrist.

Chapter 25

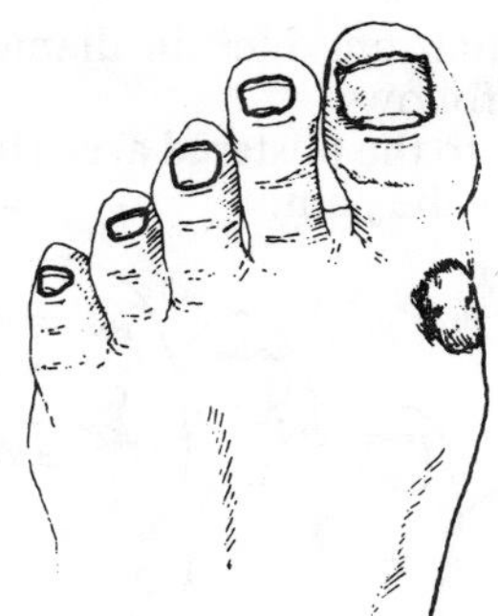

Blisters

What Are They?

A blister is an accumulation of fluid under the superficial skin surface, usually caused by excessive friction and pressure. The area around the blister is very sensitive to pressure, and continued irritation may cause redness, swelling, and eventual infection.

Things you will need for this treatment

see chapter 2 "Materials Lists" for brand names and substitutes

soap and water
antiseptic
ice bag
match
pin or needle
2"x2" gauze pads
adhesive felt or adhesive foam 1/8"
moleskin
adhesive tape ½" and 1" or 1½"
bandaids
adhesive spray and skin protectant
antibiotic cream (if you have any)
antiseptic cream
petroleum jelly
lamb's wool

Caution: *Do not proceed with this treatment until you have read the Guidelines to Treatment in Chapter 2*

Preparation for Treatment

► Make sure any instruments you use are clean. Wash them in soap and water and rinse off with alcohol or some other recognized antiseptic.

► Make sure all materials and suggested medications are clean and up to date.

► Thoroughly scrub the entire foot with warm soapy water and a terry wash cloth. Pat dry with a soft clean towel.

► Read through all the instructions which follow, and make sure you understand them before beginning treatment.

Treatment

If the blister is less than one inch in diameter and you are in no pain, leave it alone. Otherwise proceed as follows:

1. Apply an ice pack to the blistered area (for up to five minutes). This will provide some numbness and alleviate the pain.

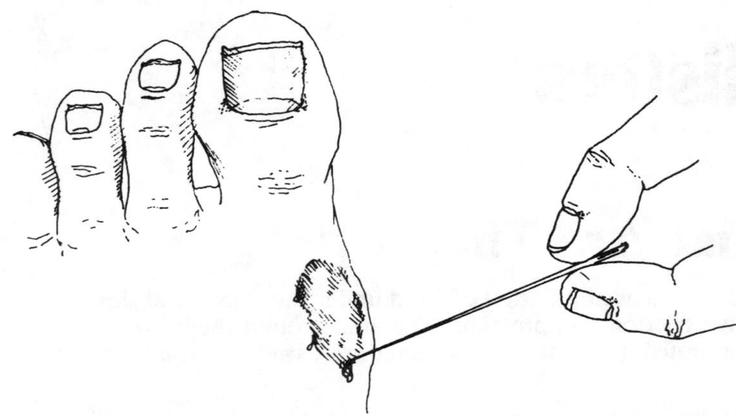

2. To drain the blister, puncture it in several places around its outer edges with a sterile pin or the tip of a scissor. (to sterilize the pin or scissor tip, either place a lighted match to it or dip it in alcohol.)

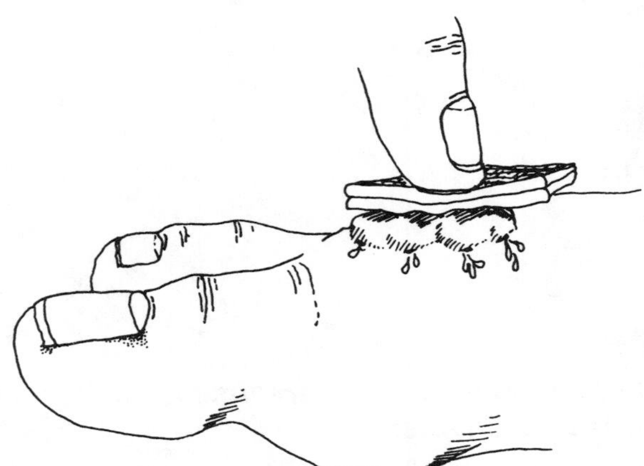

3. Squeeze the fluid out of the sides by applying gentle pressure to the top of the blister with your finger.

4. Leave the roof intact, and after several hours (or when the blister has filled with fluid again), repeat step #2. Continue to repeat once a day as required.

5. If the blister occurs under a callous, use the same procedure as described in step 2.
   - ► Penetrate your puncture needle through the callous itself.
   - ► Keep the callous filed down and under control after the blister has cleared up.
   - ► See chapters 8 and 9.

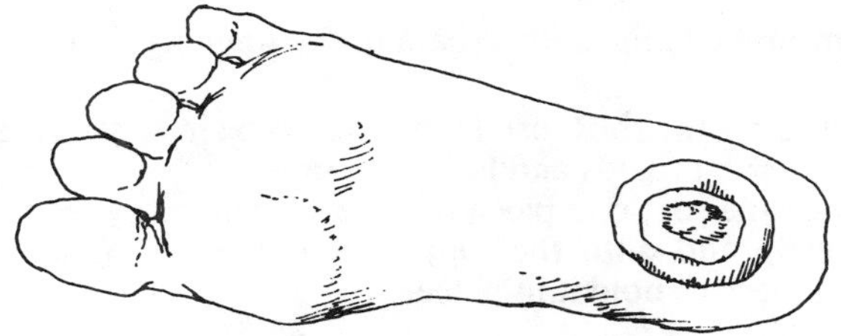

6. For blisters on the bottom of the feet (see chapters 8 and 9 for padding procedure):
   ► Using 1/8" adhesive felt or foam, cut a hole slightly larger than the blister.

   ► The remaining circle of padding (outer diameter minus inner diameter) should be between ¼ and ½ inch in width.

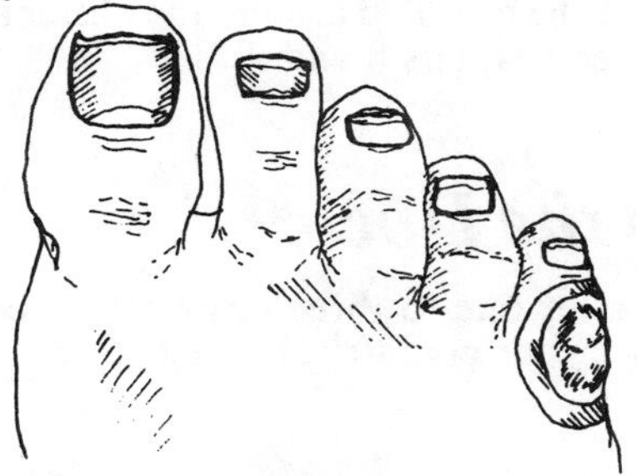

   ► Place pad on skin surrounding the blister.

7. For toe blisters:
   ► Cut a hole in a piece of moleskin slightly larger than the blister.
   ► The remaining circle of padding should be between ¼ and ½ inch in width (outer diameter minus inner diameter).
   ► Place pad on skin surrounding the blister.

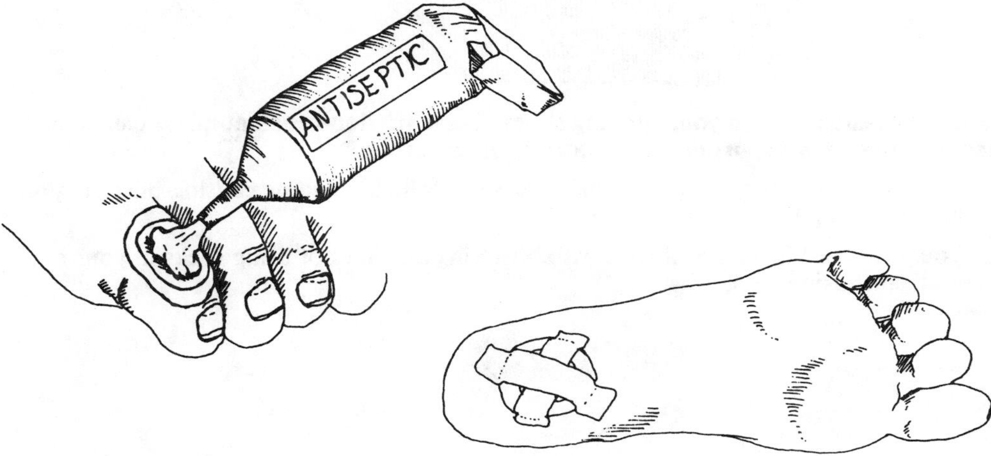

8. Put a liberal amount of antiseptic cream in the opening. Cover with sterile gauze and tape down.

► For the bottom of the foot, use 1" or 1½" tape in criss-cross fashion.
► For the toes, use bandaids and half-inch tape.
► For the tip of the toe, one piece of tape or bandaid goes from the bottom of the toe around the tip and onto the top; a second piece of tape or bandaid is placed around the first piece to hold it in place.

9. To help the tape adhere better, spray the skin first with tincture of Benzoin.

10. If you want to continue running until the blister is healed, apply a liberal amount of vaseline over the blistered area.

► For the toes: After the VASELINE™, cover the toes with lamb's wool or criss-crossed bandaids with the gauze pads over the nail plates.
► For the bottom of the feet: Pad around the blister as described earlier in the treatment and tape it down (see chapters 8 and 9).

When to Call the Doctor

If pain is not reduced after one to three days, or if you see any signs of heat, redness, swelling, or infection, see your podiatrist immediately.

Practical Pointers for Prevention

1. For toe blisters, see the running shoe section of the the appendix on shoes, for information on how to increase the forefoot and toe space of running shoes and to alleviate the pressure of the shoes on the toes.

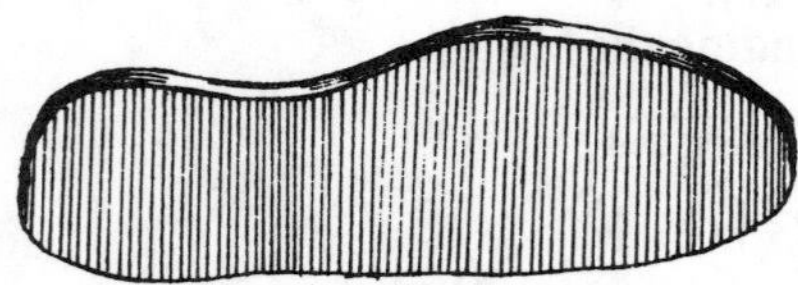

2. Place a Spenco inlay in your running shoes. These friction-resistant inlays can be purchased in your size in a sporting goods store or drug store.

3. Check your shoes for any rough seams or spots which could be causing blistering on the inside of the uppers.

4. If you have been having problems with blistering and are not using socks in your running shoes, start using them now.

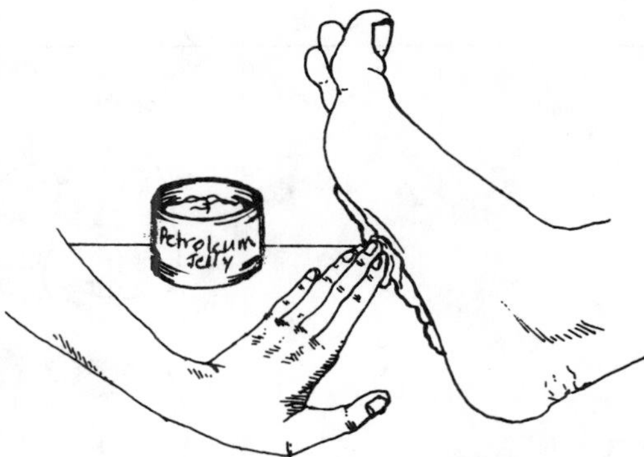

5. Before a long run or a race, especially in hot or inclement weather, apply a handful of VASELINE™ to the entire bottom of the foot. Put a ped or running sock over it, and you will have a good friction-resistant surface. The use of powder can also be effective here.

6. Always wear clean white socks. The best kind is 100% cotton or a cotton and wool blend.

7. If you wear inlays, orthotics, heel cups, etc., be sure that they are properly placed in the shoes.

8. If you are wearing new running shoes, be sure that they have been broken in properly. Walk around with them for several days before attempting to run in them, and then use them initially only on shorter runs.

DON'TS

- Don't remove the roof of the blister. Always leave the roof on.
- Don't use crinkled, soiled, or damp socks.
- Don't use tube socks that fit several sizes.
- Don't start runs in shoes that are wet from a previous run.

Chapter 26

Pain in Ball of Foot

(Dancer's Foot)

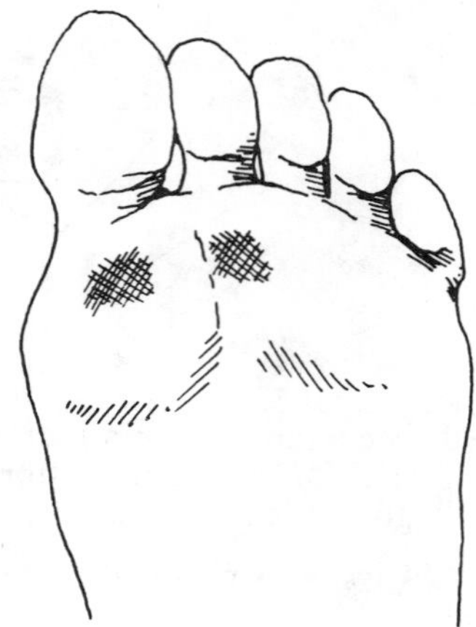

What is it?

"Dancer's Foot" is the name given to localized pain in any one of several areas on the ball of the foot corresponding to the heads of the metatarsal bones. The most common locations are under the head of the second metatarsal bone behind the second toe area, and under the first metatarsal head (sesamoid or accessory bone area) just behind the big toe.

Things you will need for this treatment

see chapter 2 "Materials List" for brand names and substitutes

soap & water
ice bag
adhesive spray and skin protectant
adhesive foam or felt 1/8" and ¼"
adhesive tape ½"
nitrogen-impregnated foam innersoles
aspirin

Caution: *Do not proceed with this treatment until you have read the Guidelines to Treatment in Chapter 2*

Treatment

1. Apply ice for five to ten minutes at the end of the day or after athletic activity. Repeat icing two to three times a day during the acute stage.

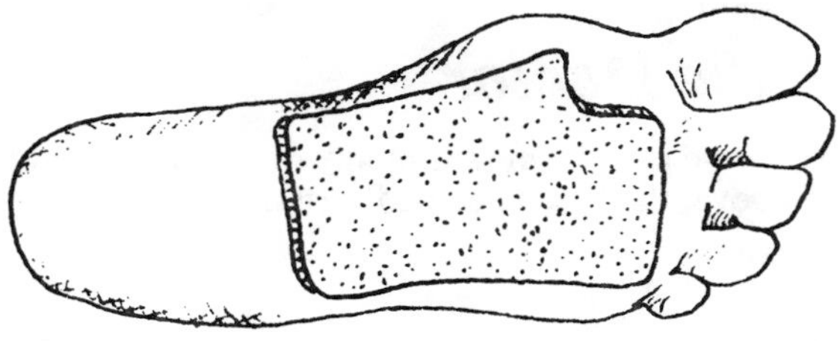

2. During the acute stage, make a pad out of 1/8" or 1/4" felt to remove the pressure from the painful spot. For more detailed instructions on making a pad, see chapter 8.

3. Take two aspirin every four hours for two days, and two aspirin every six hours for up to seven days after that.

4. If the pain is so severe that you are having difficulty participating in sports or even walking, get off your feet and rest the area as much as possible. During this time, keep the area padded to protect it from the pressure of any unavoidable walking.

After you are ready to resume athletic activities...

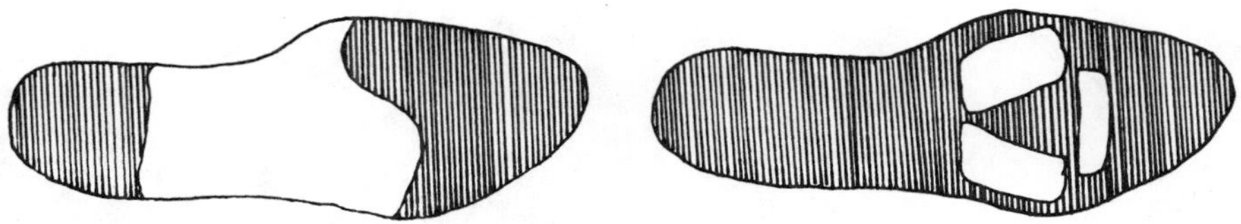

1. Place the padding on a Spenco inlay instead of directly on your foot, so that you can have extra protection while running that you may not need at other times.

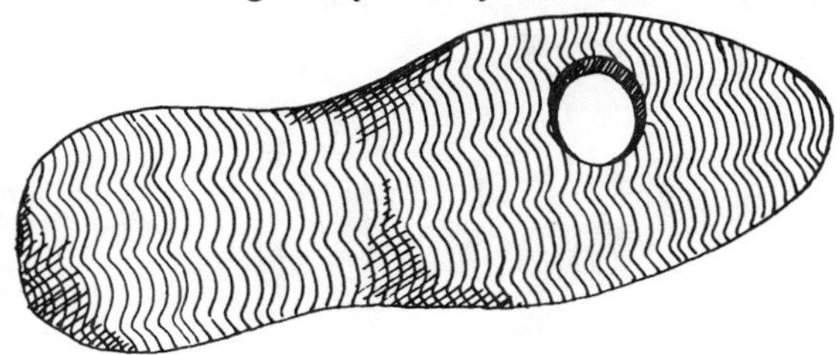

2. Make sure your athletic shoes have good forefoot shock absorption and flexibility. If you are a runner and your ball-of-foot pain is chronic, cut a portion of the sole out of your running shoe to create a depression that will keep the weight off the painful area. This can also be done to most walking shoes. The best type of shoe to use for this condition is a ripple sole.

3. If you are a runner, avoid speed workouts, racing or running on your toes or the balls of your feet. If you prefer to run on the balls of your feet, then add a heel raise made out of ¼" felt thinned down toward the front. The heel raise can be either inserted directly in your running shoes or attached to the bottom of a Spenco inlay (see appendix on Shoe Inserts You Can Make).

4. Do not wear racing shoes until the pain has disappeared.

5. If you are a dancer or gymnast and cannot or prefer not to use inserts, use a dancer's pad taped directly to your foot (see chapter 8).

When to Call the Doctor

If severe swelling or excessive pain is present in any of the injured areas after four days of treatment as described above, then see your podiatrist.

DON'TS

- **Don't wear high-heeled shoes.**
- **Don't wear exercise sandals.**
- **Don't walk barefoot.**

Chapter 27

Bump on Top of Foot

(Dorsal exostosis)

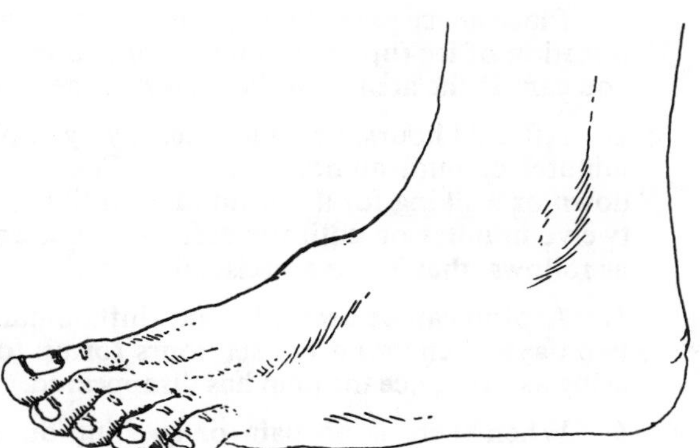

What is it?

A dorsal exostosis is a bony enlargement on top of the foot which can often become irritated and painful.

Caution: ***Do not proceed with this treatment until you have read the Guidelines to Treatment in Chapter 2***

Things you will need for this treatment

see chapter 2 "Materials List" for brand names and substitutes

soap & water
ice bag
aspirin
moleskin
adhesive foam 1/8"
petroleum jelly
2"x2" gauze pads
adhesive tape 1½"
adhesive felt ¼"
nitrogen-impregnated foam innersoles
adhesive spray and skin protectant

Preparation for Treatment

1. **Make sure all the materials and medications you will be using are clean and fresh as discussed in chapter 2.**

2. **Read through all the instructions which follow, and make sure you understand them before beginning treatment.**

3. **Thoroughly scrub the entire foot with warm soapy water and a terry wash cloth. Pat dry with a soft clean towel.**

Treatment

1. Place an ice pack directly over the painful area for up to 30 minutes. Continue the application of ice (up to 30 minutes on, 30 minutes off) for as much of the first 24 hours as you can. If the area is swollen, elevate the foot on two pillows while applying the ice pack.

2. After 24 hours, begin ice therapy by applying ice on the bumpy area for six to twelve minutes or until numbness ensues. Then actively exercise the foot by moving it up and down or walking for a few minutes until the pain returns. Then repeat the icing for six to twelve minutes or until the area is numb, and exercise again. Repeat this entire process as follows (that is, *ice*-exercise; *ice*-exercise; *ice*).

3. Aspirin can be useful for anti-inflammatory purposes. Take two every four hours for two days, then two every six hours for up to a week (see precautions in chapter 2). Stop using aspirin once the pain has disappeared.

4. When there is no pain or swelling during walking, you are ready to resume your athletic activities.

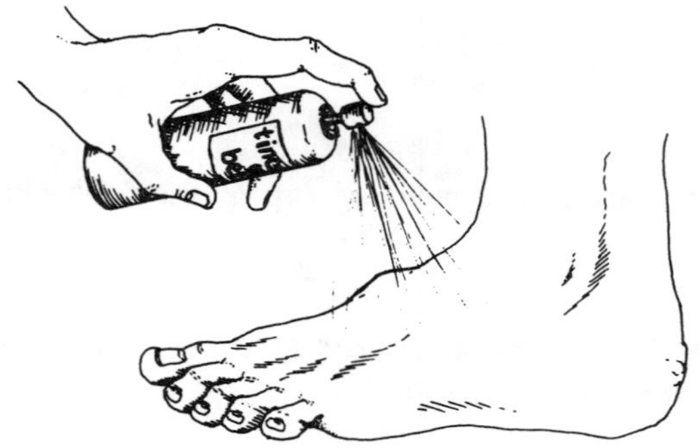

5. To protect the area from further irritation, spray tincture of Benzoin on the area to be taped.

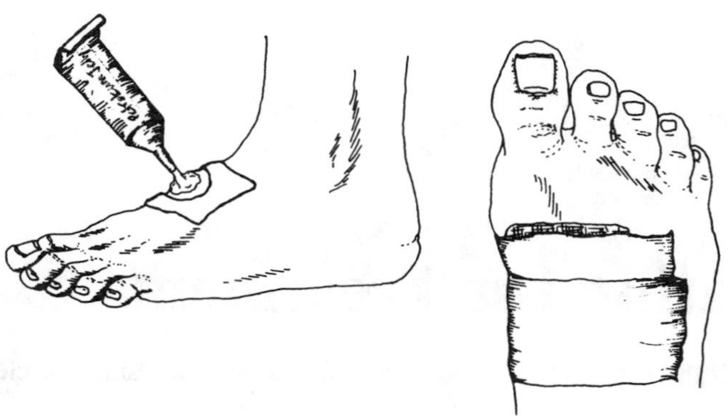

6. Cut a hole in a piece of moleskin or ⅛″ foam and place it around the bump. Remember to make the hole slightly larger than the bump itself. The remaining circle of padding should be between ¼″ and ½″ in width around the bump. Put VASELINE™ on the bump and tape a 2×2 gauze pad over the circle.

7. If pain or swelling returns after a day or two, repeat the ice treatment and rest the foot from athletic activity for a day.

8. If the pain actually makes you limp or interferes with your running form, or if severe swelling occurs, then take two to seven days off with ice therapy daily and aspirin. Pad as above to relieve the pressure on walking and pad the back of the tongue on all of your shoes. Take 1/8'' foam or several layers of moleskin and adhere to the inside of the tongue of the shoe (see chapter 21, treatment#10.

DON'TS

1. Don't lace your shoes too tightly.
2. Don't put tape on too tightly.
3. Don't run if there is severe swelling, pain, or limping.

Practical Pointers for Prevention

1. If you are very flat-footed or pronate (roll inward at the ankle) too much, or if you are severely bow-legged and have excessive heel wear on the outsides of your running shoes, try using either a varus wedge in the shoe or a Spenco inlay with a varus wedge attached. If you are flatfooted, an arch wedge also should be used. See the appendix on Shoe Inserts You Can Make.

2. The lacing of the shoe may be a cause of irritation to the bump on top of the foot, leading to excessive pressure. If so, use 1/8'' foam or several layers of moleskin on the inside of the tongue of the shoe. See illustration above.

3. To reduce irritation, use an extra pair of socks.

When to Call the Doctor

If, after several days of treatment, there is persistent heat, redness, swelling, or severe pain, see a podiatrist.

Chapter 28

Pregnancy and Foot Care

Certain foot and leg changes are considered normal during this special period of a woman's life. Lower-leg fatigue, sudden cramping and feeling of heaviness in the legs, varicose veins, and swelling of the feet and legs are the more common changes. One or more of these will usually occur and should disappear after the birth of the child. Varicose veins will often disappear as well.

Because of the increased weight and swelling of the feet, certain foot problems that were dormant can become painful now. Common foot problems such as corns, calluses, ingrown nails, warts, etc., should be taken care of if they cause pain. See the appropriate chapter or chapters pertaining to each one.

If you ignore these problems or walk around with pain, you may adapt to a way of walking that causes instability in your gait, thus risking an unnecessary fall or sprained ankle. If you compensate enough, you could wind up with a sciatica problem or unnecessary backache. Therefore, take care of foot problems as soon as you notice them. You will eliminate unnecessary fatigue and skeletal system discomfort and decrease the possibility that an unusual gait pattern or stance will exert excessive strain on the muscles, ligaments, and bones.

Footwear During Pregnancy

Continued normal activities and exercises are recommended during pregnancy, but appropriate footwear is vital. This is not the time for high heels, pointed shoes, or loose, floppy non-supportive casual ones.

1. Proper shoes are crepe-soled wedgies, similar to nurse or waitress shoes.

2. The uppers should be good supportive material like leather and the heel heighth should be an inch and one-half or less.

3. Generally, the lowest shoe with the widest heel and broadest, toe-box area that you can become accustomed to physically and mentally is the best.

Hints About Heels

Many women are used to wearing stylish shoes with high, narrow heels and narrow toes. Aside from the instability these shoes naturally cause, if one's feet are to swell, unnecessary problems can occur during pregnancy.

1. If you have worn high-heeled shoes for many years, your calf muscles may have shortened and the lower heeled shoe will cause you discomfort. Early in the pregnancy it is a good idea to gradually decrease the heel heighth of your daily shoe, so that later on you will be able to wear shoes that will afford you the most comfort and stability.

2. Your goal is to wear shoes with an inch-and-a-half heel heighth or less.

3. Decrease heel heighth one-quarter inch every four weeks if you wear shoes with heel heighths of higher than one-and-a-half inches.

4. You might try wearing a walking or running shoe around the house. If this is too uncomfortable at first, add a one-quarter inch to one-half inch heel raise inside the shoe. (See "Shoe inserts you can make" for details.) Eventually, you should be able to eliminate the heel lift.

5. Start doing calf-stretching exercises once or twice a day.

Shoe Shopping Tips

1. When buying shoes, your feet will probably be swollen, especially in humid weather. To get a proper fit, make sure that you have room across the ball of your foot. You should be able to pinch up the leather or other material.

2. Be sure to buy shoes in the evening or when the swelling is greatest.

3. You may even have to wear two different size widths or styles if you have periods of excessive swelling.

4. To allow for swelling at certain periods you can probably get one pair of shoes that should last the entire pregnancy by having them filled with an extra innersole They will still fit when your feet go down to their normal size. As your feet get larger, just remove the innersoles.

5. See appendix C—Shoes.

6. All leather shoes are much better than synthetics as far as breatheability and flexibility. Also, synthetic heels are more slippery. If you do have such a pair, change the heel to one made out of rubber.

7. If your heels wear out too quickly, replace them or get new shoes to keep yourself from twisting your ankles.

8. Do not wear slippers, moccasins, or thongs, and you shouldn't go barefooted around the house. You need the support of tennis, running, or good walking shoes.

9. Do not wear clogs at all. They can lead to too many injuries.

10. Many women participate in fitness activities nowadays and are often encouraged to do so by their obstetricians during their pregnancies. Be sure to wear the appropriate shoes for the athletic activity you are involved in, such as a tennis shoe for tennis or a running shoe for running. Watch your normal shoe size here. To allow for swelling, you may have to get a larger shoe size or a second pair of shoes with an innersole as described previously. See appendix C—Shoes.

11. Because of the extra weight and stress on the feet and legs, the feet may begin to burn, especially the ball of the feet. If this occurs, purchase a friction-resistant shock-absorbing innersole like a Spenco inlay, Scholl's innersole or similar product. They come in all shoe sizes and will help alleviate the above problems.

Looking Out for Yourself

1. Most of use are born with inherent foot and leg structural weaknesses that can lead to various foot and postural problems. With the additional stress due to the extra weight, some of these heretofore dormant problems may become symptomatic. If this occurs, read over appendix B—Foot Structure and Function. Then see appendix D—Shoe Inserts You Can Make.

2. You should try to avoid accidents that could cause inconvenience and unnecessary pain. Do not walk around barefooted at night—you certainly do not need the added burden of a fractured toe or two because you stubbed your toe walking into something you couldn't see.

3. Do not wear improperly fitting or constrictive hosiery. Make sure you have enough room for toe motion. Ask your obstetrician for advice on types of supportive hose. Do not get the regular support hose, which are often too restrictive and may not fit you well enough. You should purchase toeless and heelless surgical stockings that are elastic and supportive with a lot of room for the toes. They can be worn under your regular nylon stockings and are available at surgical supply houses. The best ones are made specifically to your measurements.

4. If your feet swell excessively, are tired, cramping, or feel heavy, elevate them on two pillows and wiggle your toes gently for short periods of time or as often as you can.

5. Gently massage your feet and legs or have them massaged using baby oil or massage lotion to reduce friction, five to ten minutes once or twice daily.

6. Purchase a "Footsie Roller"™ for your feet and use a vibrator for your legs.

7. Do the following series of exercises while lying down in bed once or twice daily: (consult chapter 30).

- The inversion-eversion exercise.
- Plantar-flexion-dorsi-flexion.
- Ankle circling.
- Toe exercises.
- Sometimes the feet perspire excessively during this period of your life. If this is so, consult chapter 13, "Sweaty and Smelly Feet."

8. Also, ankle- or knee-high socks are often held in place by elastic garter-like bands. Be careful that they are not too constrictive for your legs and circulation. If they are, try a larger size or do not use them at all.

9. Every once in a while examine your legs for varicose veins. If these red spider-like network of veins occur, support elastic stockings may be helpful. Consult your obstetrician.

10. Good basic general rules for foot health should also be followed.

    A. Keep your feet clean.

    B. Wash them daily with soap and water.

    C. Dry them thoroughly, especially between the toes, and do not rub with a coarse towel.

D. Apply lubricating cream to the feet such as vegetable shortening, cocoa butter, vitamin A Cream, or a mixture of fifty percent Crisco oil liquid and fifty percent VASELINE,™ etc.

E. Cut the toenails straight across.

Chapter 29

Children's Problems

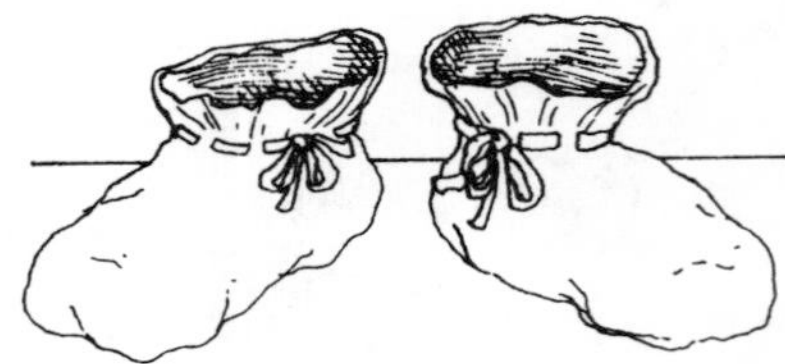

Children's foot problems can appear at early ages. In many cases the children do not even know they have problems and don't complain about them. It is very important for parents to examine for early developmental problems. Many deformities can be detected and more serious ones prevented by early recognition. These are often hereditary in nature and if present in the parents and grandparents, an early examination of your child is even more important.

Unfortunately, many parents are mistakenly told by other professionals, relatives, and friends that certain foot and leg positions or pains are to be ignored as the child will most likely outgrow them. Most often this is not true and by the time a podiatrist sees the child, treatment has to be geared toward compensating for a problem that the person is going to have to live with. It is too late for a cure. The sooner the problem is recognized and dealt with, the faster it can be resolved. Certain positions, walking patterns and foot and leg configurations may look strange, however, in a particular age group they may be considered normal and should be outgrown.

This section attempts to help you identify the different problems you may encounter in your children. After reading this chapter you will be able to determine whether the advice you've gotten from professionals or friends is accurate, or whether your child should be checked further by a specialist such as a podiatrist.

Babies

Babies do not need shoes or socks until they can stand and/or begin to walk. Any foot coverings should be *loose* and provide warmth. Use non-stretch cotton socks approximately two sizes larger than indicated to allow extra room for the toes to wiggle. You can also use a baby garment with feet and legs, but be careful about shrinkage after laundering. The sole should be flexible if you are going to use booties. Don't forget that babies quickly outgrow clothes. Check the length and fit every time you put them on the baby.

No binding bed covers should be placed over the child's feet. They can retard development by not allowing the child freedom to exercise the feet and legs. This is important as they prepare for walking. If you insist on covering up the child, tuck a roll of diapers, a towel, or a cover at the foot of the crib under the covers to keep them held loosely over the baby's feet.

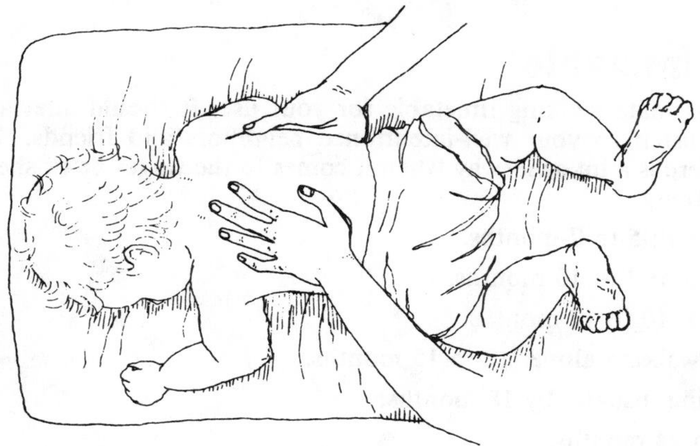

Change the baby's lying position several times each day, Prolonged time in one position, especially on the stomach, can put excessive strain on the foot and leg. To get the child onto his side while sleeping, put a roll of diapers, a towel, or rolled-up blanket next to him to prevent the child from rolling over onto his stomach. Or, put a roll next to the child's back and anchor it against the side of the crib.

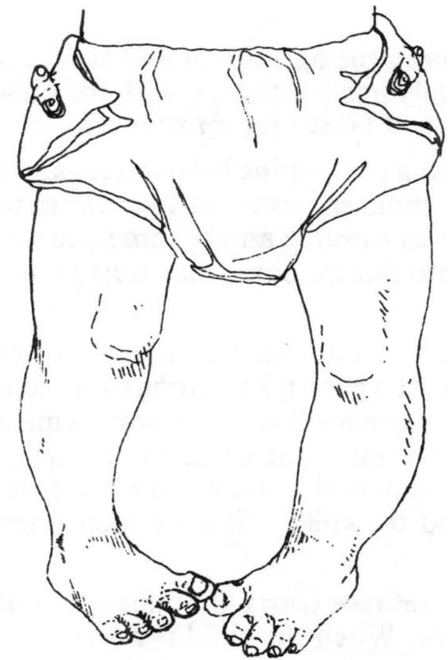

Too many layers of diapers can sometimes cause the child to assume a bow-legged-like position. More than a double layer is unnecessary unless there is a specific reason. For example, your podiatrist may suggest this to correct a knock-kneed positional problem.

Do not rush a child to walk. Do not compare your child to any other children. The average walking age is between ten and eighteen months, but there are large differences among individuals. Definitely do not pressure the child to walk by holding him or her by the armpits or putting the child in a walker, forcing the feet to dangle in order to hasten the process. It won't work and could possibly cause muscle injury and strain.

Walking Timetable

Here is an approximate walking timetable for your use. It should alleviate some of your anxieties. Don't listen to your well-intentioned neighbors and friends. *Your* child is an individual and there is a lot of leeway when it comes to the stages he or she will go through from birth to walking.

- Attempts to crawl; 5 to 7 months.
- Attempts to stand: 7 to 10 months.
- Ability to stand: 10 to 12 months.
- Confidence in walking alone: 12 to 15 months.
- Adept at walking: usually by 18 months.
- Running: 20 to 24 months.
- Running, jumping, and feeling totally secure in their ability to do this: by 3 years old.

(If a child is a bit overweight, these time tables may be slowed down even more.)

Steps Toward Walking

1. The first steps come anywhere between seven to eighteen months, but the average is ten to eighteen months.

2. Children will usually sit up between the ages seven and twelve months, with the average being seven to nine months. This really has a lot to do with the child's energy level and size. Outgoing children and lightweights will be sitting up sooner.

3. The child will usually start crawling or creeping between six and twelve months. Crawling usually begins at six months. Some children never really crawl much before walking; many children who crawl earlier may use it as a crutch and become late walkers. Other children are clumsy crawlers and keep banging into things. Some may hurt themselves so much it actually hastens their drive to learn to walk.

4. The child may stand alone by seven months, but anywhere between seven and sixteen months can be considered normal; it may even take as long as eighteen months. The child first stands holding on with both hands, then eventually using one hand and then none. Often the child doesn't even realize what he or she has done when on his own for the first time. Walking occurs when the child is physically and mentally ready and not before. Do not push your child. This can often lead to resistance and the child will walk later rather than when he is really ready.

   A. Parents of early walkers sometimes worry that this could be damaging to the child's feet and legs. This is not really so. When the child is ready to walk, he or she will walk. Some do so earlier than others.

   B. Sometimes a child is bow-legged or knock-kneed when he first starts to walk and this can happen with both early and late walkers.

5. Once the child begins to walk, there is a simple "trick" you can do to the playpen if you use it quite a bit. Take a blanket that is big enough to tuck under the playpen mattress. Tucking the blanket in not only helps keep the child's feet warm but also helps provide some resilience and enables the child to better grasp the surface, easing the transition to walking.

6. Certain factors can influence a child's walking habits even when there is nothing physically wrong with the child's feet or legs.

A. Children are great imitators. They will copy postural habits of adults or other children around them such as turning their feet in or out, limping, and stooping.

B. Dance positions where the feet are turned out and very wide-spread legs are often signs of poor balance. If the child is encouraged to walk before he is ready, these conditions may develop into fixed positions and actual problems can occur. Again, when the child is physically and emotionally ready to walk, he will walk. Don't compare your children to anyone else's. Excessive parental guidance may be injurious to the child.

C. Always putting the child to sleep on his stomach or in a frog leg position can cause spread leg positions.

D. Certain toys can lead to muscular imbalance between the body's two sides. (For example, toys like scooters cause the child to favor one leg over the other.)

E. Improper diet and nutrition can often lead to weakened, underdeveloped muscles. It can also cause poor posture, leading to poor walking habits.

F. Unhappy, frightened, and tense children often have their muscles under constant tension and this can cause problems. Shy children have shown they can develop feelings of inferiority and become depressed. Depressed children can have poor posture or poor walking habits.

7. At some point between seven and eighteen months, the child will begin to walk.

A. A child's feet may appear flat for a long period of time. This is not necessarily abnormal, and is due to a fat pad in the arch that disappears between the ages of two and one-half to three. If the foot appears flat after age three, have it checked by a doctor.

B. Children usually start to walk with their feet turned outward to gain stability. This eventually straightens out.

C. If the child starts to walk with the feet straight ahead, they are likely to end up toeing-in. This is considered abnormal and should be checked by a podiatrist.

D. A child will normally waddle and seem to be almost running—to "fall" from step to step.

E. The knees should be bent slightly.

F. The feet and legs should be turned outward.

G. The hands are usually in the air with the arms held out for added stability.

H. The child's motions actually look very clumsy, like a series of forward falls.

I. In time, the child will develop confidence. This early clumsiness should disappear by eighteen to twenty months of age.

Children's Examination

Here is a 12-part examination that you can perform with your own child, to determine whether there are any structural weaknesses present. Many problems with children's feet, legs, hips, and back may be avoided by early recognition and proper attention. Youngsters will seldom realize or tell you that what they are experiencing is painful or bad for them. It is up to you to watch them and check periodically for signs of trouble. Improper foot and leg structure can lead to many problems that extend through adolescence and into adult life.

1. Watch your child walk and run.
   - Does he like or dislike it or complain about it?

- **Does the walk seem peculiar?**
- **Does the child stumble or fall down excessively?**
- **Does the child always take his or her shoes off?**

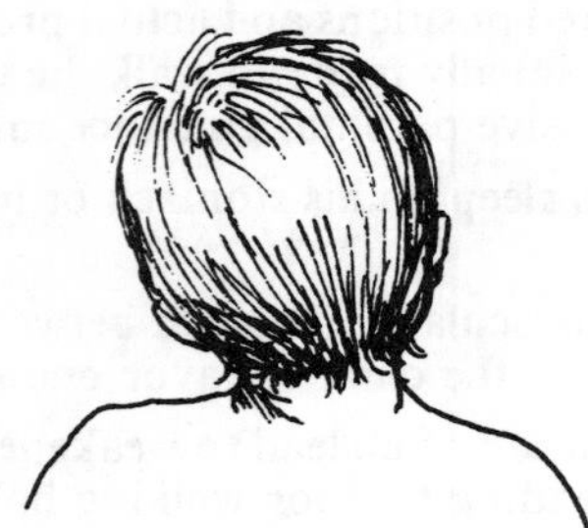

- **Does the head usually tilt to one side or another?**
- **Is one shoulder lower than the other? (See appendix on Foot Structure and Function.)**
- **Do the hips seem to be level? (See appendix on Foot Structure and Function.)**
- **Does one arm swing lower than the other?**

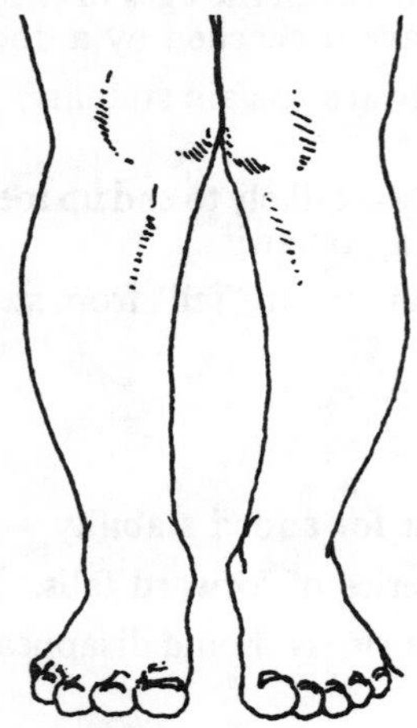

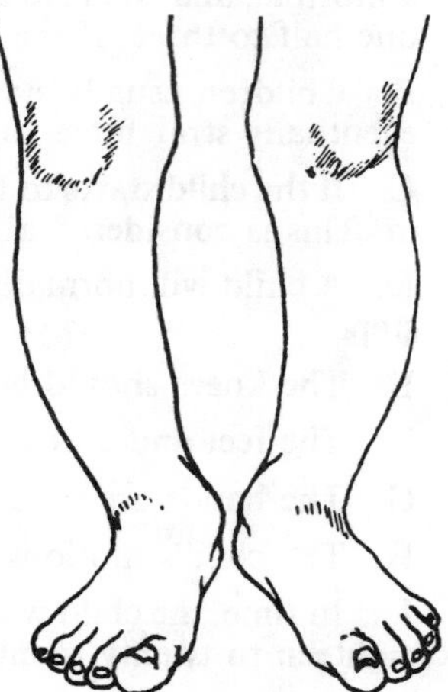

- **Do the knees seem to be pointed inward or outward rather than straight ahead?**
- **Do the feet turn in or out when the child stands?**
- **Do the feet turn in or out when the child walks?**

Toeing-Out

Slight toeing-out can be normal up to three years of age. As the child first begins to walk, the feet normally turn out to try to give the child a sense of equilibrium. Once this is reached, the feet gradually straighten out and are positioned closer together and more parallel. By the time the child is four years old the toeing-out should completely disappear. If the child toes-out excessively he should be treated.

If it goes untreated, this condition can often lead to awkward gait, poor posture, excessive fatigue, lower back pain, leg pains, and leg cramping.

Toeing-In

Toeing-in or a pigeon-toed gait (walking) is the most common foot condition seen in children. It should not be present after the child is adept at walking. At best, the child's feet should be straight or toed-out slightly. If, however, the child's feet are turned in, consult a podiatrist.

1. Does the child toe-walk?
This usually means that there are shortened muscles in the back of the leg, which could lead to leg and back problems in adulthood.

2. Does the child limp?
There are many reasons for limping. Whether or not the child complains about a limp, it should be checked out.

There is something called a "ten-day limp," where a child will limp for ten days for no known reason and then stop. If you have to wait to get it checked and you're worried about it, don't lose too much sleep over it. Chances are it's not serious.

3. Does the child lift his heels off the ground too quickly (premature heel lift)?
The ramifications of this are similar to toe-walking.

4. Does the child complain of night cramps? (Does he or she wake up in the middle of the night with cramping or muscle spasms in the legs?)
This should not occur. There is no such thing as "growing pains." This is an indication that the child's leg muscles are fatigued and often indicates foot and leg structural weakness. It can also be due to other conditions but these are less likely. (See chapter 24—Cramps.)

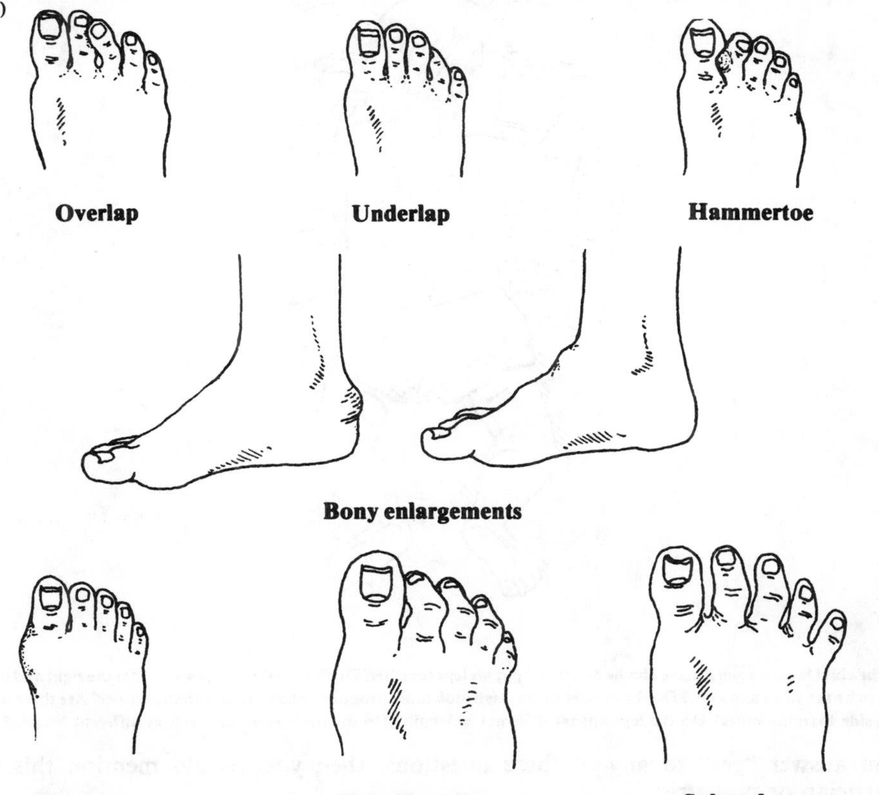

5. Have your child stand. When you put the ankles together, do the knees touch first? Is there space between the ankles? (Are the legs knock-kneed?) (See appendix B—Foot Structure and Function.)

When the ankles are together, is there a wide space between the knees (bowed legs)? (See appendix B—Foot Structure and Function.)

Knocked-knees and bowed-legs are common problems as the child develops his sense of balance. They should disappear as the child develops more security in his or her walking habits. Bowed-legs are considered normal up to at least eighteen months of age. The legs should straighten out after three years. Knocked-knees, however, may not completely disappear until the child is somewhere between three and six years of age.

6. Do the child's arches appear very flat or very high? (See appendix B—Foot Structure and Function.)

7. Does the child have a "C" shaped foot? This type of foot means that the bones inside the feet under the skin are turned inward too much. This condition is called *metatarsus adductus,* and should have been treated already. If the child stands and starts to walk like this, a professional consultation is indicated as soon as possible.

8. Ask the child to turn around with his back to you. Do the tendons in the back of the lower leg bow outward? (See appendix B—Foot Structure and Function.)

9. Have the child sit down and take his shoes off. Does one toe overlap another? Does one toe underlap another? Are there any hammertoes, bunions, or bony enlargements on the back of the heel or on top of the foot? Are the toes claw-like when the child stands? Do the feet splay out with the toes wide apart and look very loose?

10. Sometimes babies are born with two toes connected by a thin skin membrane. This is called webbed-toes. Parents can become alarmed about this but it is a harmless condition that will not interfere with the baby's walking. Webbed-toes are not usually noticed later in life. The only treatment for this is corrective surgery which we feel is unnecessary except for cosmetic purposes.

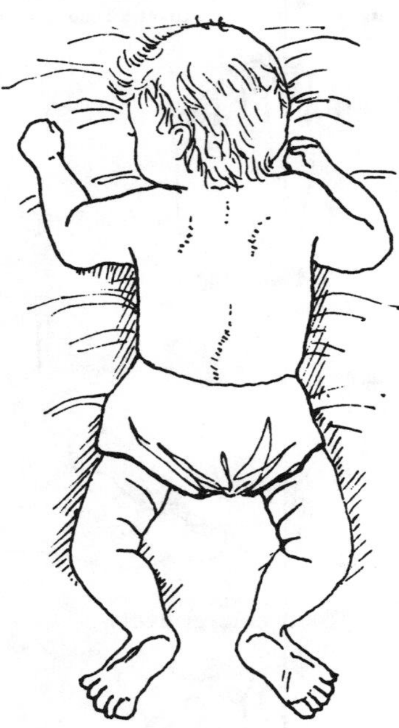

11. If the child is very young, have him lie down and put his legs together. Do the number of creases under the right and left buttocks appear to be the same and even? Do the creases in the thigh look more pronounced on one side than another? Are there more creases on one side than the other? Do the legs appear different in length? Do the heels seem to touch at different lengths?

If you answer "yes" to any of these questions, then you should mention this to your pediatrician or podiatrist.

12. Children may not complain about their feet, but check the following:
   - Do the feet perspire too much?
   - Are there any infections, blisters, or areas of redness?
   - Are there any rashes?
   - Are there any unusual growths?
   - Is there any redness or pain around the toenails?
   - Does the child complain of pain anywhere in the feet?
   - Is there bad posture?
   - Do the child's shoes wear out unevenly and run down peculiarly on one side?

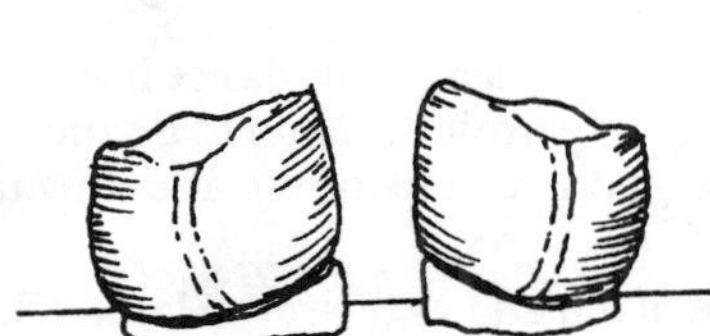

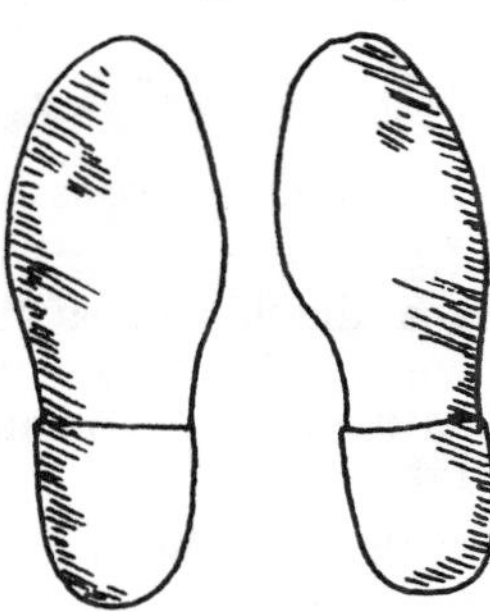

   - Does the child usually get tired and cranky easily? Does he complain of pains in other parts of his body, (back, neck, or hip) after playing or standing for long periods of time? Does he like to play?
   - Does the child always seem to want to sit down a lot?

If the answers to any of these questions are "yes," see a podiatrist or have your pediatrician refer you to a podiatrist.

Finally, for questions concerning children's shoes, see appendix C—Shoes.

What To Remember When Your Child Goes To The Doctor

1. Many children outgrow the problems that are present at specific ages. For example, certain conditions that may be a problem at ages five, six, or seven may be normal at age two or vice versa.

2. Treating the problem is just the beginning of the therapy. Many times it takes years of cooperation between child, parent, and doctor in order to alleviate particular conditions. It is important to realize that once correction is achieved, no matter how it is arrived at, it may take a very long period of time to maintain the correction. Therefore, you must have patience and work together as a team.

3. As an informal rule of thumb, remember that for every year a condition goes untreated, it takes about two years to either correct it or compensate for it.

4. When the parents and child enter the room with the doctor, let the child do as much talking as his or her age permits. There are certain things that children may tell the doctor that

they may not even tell you. Help them if you have to but try to stay out of the way as much as possible unless the doctor asks for your cooperation.

5. Some of the foot treatments a doctor may utilize are paddings, tapings, strappings, plaster immobilization, taking plaster prints, shoe accommodations, or variations and exercises. In addition, special inlays may be made (orthotics or heel stabilizers) and special activities such as ballet and ice skating may be recommended.

6. Be suspicious of and question a doctor who directs you to a laboratory to have inlays made or sends you to a shoe store to get shoes and then never asks or checks with you to see what it is you bought.

7. Rarely do shoes correct foot disorders in anyone, especially children. Shoes are basically a protective covering and if improperly fitted can aggravate certain pre-existing conditions.

Ballet and Skating: Are They Good For Your Child?

Ballet lessons and other dance lessons are often considered excellent exercise for children and can also be used as an adjunctive treatment in certain disorders.

1. It's important that the child be taught by a reputable and knowledgeable dance instructor. This teacher must come highly recommended and know not to permit the child to do toe work until the child is mature enough to handle it. If done too soon various physical deformities could result.

2. Toe dancing should be learned no sooner than the age of ten and maybe even later. Check with your community dance instructors, a University ballet association, or a national ballet company to recommend teachers in your area.

You also might consult a sports medicine podiatrist who may work with a ballet school for recommendations.

3. Roller skating and ice skating are often adjuncts to treatment of flat foot and toe-in problems in children. If your child is interested in any of these sports and you have any questions about them, consult your podiatrist. If your child is undergoing any treatment with this doctor, bring up the fact that your child would like to participate in some of these activities and find out which positions or exercises can be helpful and / or harmful to the child's foot and leg condition.

Answers to Common Foot Questions

1. Are there any exercises that help the baby's feet to develop?

There is really no need for parents to do any special exercising of their child's feet. It is more important not to interfere with the developmental process and be sure that the baby's shoes and coverings allow for normal growth and movement.

2. Is going barefoot good exercise?

If we all could walk on beautiful lawns and soft, clean, sandy beaches, going barefoot would be ideal. Unfortunately, we spend most of our time walking on hard surfaces such as sidewalks and floors, so our feet really take a beating and need some support and protection. Therefore, shoes are vital to proper development as soon as children begin to walk.

3. When should you get your child shoes?

Although children really don't need shoes before they start to walk, it is good to have some covering on the feet if it is extremely cold or if there is a chance of injury in some activity. The first shoes should be very flexible and light (like a soft glove leather). They should definitely be large enough to allow for as much freedom of movement as possible.

Children's Shoes

Shoes for Babies

Babies usually don't need shoes until they really start to walk on hard surfaces. Up until that point they only need foot coverings for the first year or so for warmth. There is really no physical need for booties or soft shoes. You must make sure whatever you put on them does not restrict the feet or toe movements. (See Chapter 29, "Children's Problems.")

1. Baby's shoe should be high, with laces over the ankles to make it harder to kick off. The shoe should be hard enough to protect the soft, pliable bony structure at the front, but soft enough to be able to bend. The shoe should be made of leather.

2. Shoes and socks should be about one-half inch longer than the baby's foot and slightly wider. The size must be changed as soon as the child has outgrown them. The size may have to be changed every month or so for the first year.

3. Baby will often give signals when his shoes are too small. He will start to complain or constantly try to pull the shoes off. There could be areas of redness around the longest (not always the biggest) toe, or where the little toe presses along the side of the shoe. Signs that shoes are too small: the tips of the soles are worn on the outside and there could also be wear marks on the inside of the shoe that lead all the way up to the front.

4. A shoe that is non-supporting can cause as much trouble as one that is too small. The stresses of walking on a shoe that is non-supportive can cause skeletal discomfort, night crying, or extreme fatigue. If a toddler or youngster wants to be carried all the time, chances are his feet and legs are tired or hurting him. The fit of the shoe and the support of the shoe should be checked.

5. A child may appear to have no arch when he stands. This is not necessarily a problem. Children have fat pads in the arch area that may give the appearance of flat feet to the untrained eye.

6. If the child walks with his ankles either rolled-out or rolled-in with his feet flattened out, he should be checked by a podiatrist. Early treatment can prevent a lifetime of discomfort.

Shoes for Older Children

1. Children's shoes should be purchased in stores that specialize in children's footwear. Avoid sales people that do not seem to know much about children's shoes. Find an individual experienced in fitting children's shoes. Be sure the store has a system to check the date and size of the shoe bought at each visit (children's feet and shoe sizes should be checked every three months). If you find such a store and are satisfied, keep going there. If you do not know of such a store, ask your podiatrist or pediatrician.

2. Between the ages of one and six, the shoe size changes every four to eight weeks; between ages six to ten the shoe size changes every twelve to sixteen weeks; between ages twelve and fifteen the size changes every sixteen to twenty weeks. Do not get fitted solely by "number;" have both feet measured.

3. When dealing with young children, be sure you are really careful with the fit. Up to two sizes too small may not appear to cause much discomfort so you have to be very careful.

4. Never accept special shoe pads or inserts from a salesperson without the advice of a podiatrist.

5. Never use hand-me-down shoes. Besides probably being worn down too much, the shoes will be forcing your child's foot into another child's mold and this could lead to trouble. In addition, skin infections like athlete's foot can be spread through footwear.

6. Make sure the children are standing when they are fitted. The shoe should be about one-half inch longer than the longest toe (which may not be the large toe). There should be enough room in the toe box from top to bottom so that the child can wiggle his toes and the toes are not pressured. The heel should fit snugly and you should be able to pinch up the leather or other shoe material across the top of the shoe with your fingers.

7. The shoe should look approximately like the shape of a foot.

8. Children's shoes should be fairly flexible. Very heavy, rigid, or inflexible shoes are just not made for walking. They do not work as the child's foot works and often do not bend where they should. Tough shoes are definitely a misconception. The shoe should be sturdy and need not be expensive.

9. Contrary to popular belief (at least in the past), sneakers are good shoes for children. Today, sneakers are very flexible and made well enough to have a good deal of shock absorption and good heel counter support. In buying sneakers, make sure that the heel and collar (especially for little children) fit snugly so the shoe does not slide off.

10. Although laced oxford shoes are preferable to loafer types or moccasins for more conventional footwear, for a "normal" foot the loafer or moccasin shoe should be okay.

11. Sandals are okay as long as the straps and openings do not cause irritation.

12. Dress-up shoes for young ladies should be worn only for dress-up periods. Many are made of synthetic materials such as patent leather and don't breathe properly. Some are not flexible enough and don't give enough support. They should be used on a part-time basis only.

13. When children are involved in athletic activities, it's a good idea to have the appropriate shoe for the appropriate activity. As a rule, a good basic sneaker is okay for most activities. However, if a child is involved in soccer, then a soccer shoe should be worn, and so forth.

14. As a general rule, shoes should not have to be broken in. They should fit and feel good right away.

15. Children's feet really do grow too quickly to get shoe repairs other than new tips and heel lifts. Children's shoes should not be resoled. When the shoe is resoled it almost always becomes smaller in the process.

16. Do not attempt to dry a wet shoe near heat. This will cause the shoe to shrink. When the child comes in from rain or snow with soaked shoes, stuff some crumpled tissue or newspaper in them and put them off in the corner away from the heat. This thorough drying process may take two or three days but won't ruin the shoes.

17. It definitely makes good sense from a long-term health and money standpoint to just throw shoes out that are no longer large enough and not in good condition.

18. After the child has worn new shoes for a day or two you might want to check his or her feet to see if there are any irritated spots. Ask them if they are having any trouble. Sometimes the shoes may be too stiff, especially in the back. Roll the palm of your hand over the back of the shoe to try to soften it up and perhaps bend the shoe in the arch area to make it more flexible.

19. There is a special polish for dressy shoes called Meltonian™ polish that comes in various colors and can soften leather if the shoe is too hard or causing irritation. If you do have trouble with fit you should take the shoes back to the shoe store and have them stretched in the appropriate area. If in doubt, return them; they're not worth keeping.

20. Again, shoes do not correct. "Corrective" shoes can instead be irritants and cause trouble. If the child has any problems, don't blame it on the shoe. It may have something to do with the way they walk. Be sure to see a podiatrist.

21. Hosiery (socks and stockings) that is too small can definitely be harmful to a child's feet. At the younger ages the hose should be rounded at the toes and as close to the shape of the foot as possible. You should also be careful about shrinkage of socks, stockings, and pantyhose after washing.

Chapter 30

Foot Care for Older Adults

As we age, our bodies change. Our skin becomes wrinkled, our hair turns gray, and some may even disappear. We do not usually look forward to these changes but they are considered normal. Similarly, our feet show certain changes with age. Our nails often get thicker, our skin drier, and we seem to notice an increase in corns, callouses, hammertoes, bunions, etc. This is an inevitable result of walking on and abusing them for many years. Many of us assume that our feet, our legs, and our bodies must naturally start to ache and feel stiffer and more uncomfortable as we get older. This is not necessarily true and with some proper preventative attention our feet and legs do not have to bother us as we age.

General Foot Care

1. Wash your feet daily in mild soap and water and dry them thoroughly and gently. Be careful to clean between the toes. Do not rub the feet with a coarse towel.

2. Use clean socks and/or stockings daily.

3. Whenever it is very damp and your feet get wet, change your socks or stockings and get into dry footwear as soon as possible.

4. If your feet perspire excessively, check to see if your shoes, socks, or stockings are permitting proper ventilation. Nylon stockings can contribute to this problem with certain individuals as can shoes made with synthetic materials and composition soles other than leather. The best socks to wear are made of pure cotton, cotton and wool, or equal parts of cotton, wool, and nylon. All leather shoes with leather soles allow for best "breatheability" in footwear.

5. Use a mild dusting powder (talcum powder) on your feet or in your socks or stockings when you change them. If you have excessive perspiration and/or foot odor problems, see Chapter 13, "Sweaty and Smelly Feet."

6. Wear properly fitted shoes as well as the appropriate shoe for special activities. Invest in a pair of good walking, jogging, or running shoes for these activities. Your feet are worth it. (See appendix C—Shoes.)

7. Do not wear excessively tight socks or stockings. These are often too constrictive and can interfere with circulation and ventilation.

8. As we get older, we often encounter various foot and leg circulation problems. These are generally due to overall health states and should be brought to the attention of your physician.

However, if you've checked with your doctor and have no debilitating diseases, a regular exercise program is the most effective way to improve the circulation in your feet and legs.

The following series of simple exercises for the feet and legs should be done daily:

A. Flexion-Extension

Starting position: Sit with back straight in chair, feet six to twelve inches off floor.

Steps of Exercise:

Step 1. Move feet at ankle and bring them toward you as much as possible. Hold for three seconds.

Step 2. Move feet at ankle and point toes toward the floor as much as possible. Hold for three seconds.

Step 3. Relax for three seconds. Repeat.

Repetitions: Do a minimum of twenty times, twice daily.

B. Foot Circling

Starting position: Sit with back straight in chair, feet six to twelve inches off floor.

Steps of Exercise:

Step 1. Slowly rotate feet in clockwise direction. Continue for thirty seconds.

Step 2. Slowly rotate feet in counter-clockwise direction. Continue for thirty seconds.

Repetitions: Do a minimum of six times, twice daily.

C. Four-Step

Starting position: Sit with back straight in chair. Bend legs to right angle. Place feet several inches apart and point them straight ahead. Place feet on one inch book, toes extending over edge.

Steps of Exercise:

Step 1. Curl toes down over edge of book as much as possible. Hold for three seconds.

Step 2. Keeping feet flat on book raise toes toward ceiling as much as possible. Hold for three seconds.

Step 3. Keeping heel on book, raise feet toward shins. Hold for three seconds.

Step 4. Return feet to starting position. Repeat.

Repetitions: Do a minimum of ten times, twice daily.

D. Inversion-Eversion

Starting position: Sit with back straight in chair, feet six to twelve inches off floor, legs extended.

Steps of exercise:

Step 1. Turn feet inward and hold for three seconds.

Step 2. Turn feet outward and hold for three seconds.

Step 3. Return to starting position. Repeat.

Repetitions: Do a minimum of twenty times, twice daily.

Comments: Do not move knees during exercise.

E. Towel Pull

Starting position: Sit with back straight in chair. Bend legs to right angle. Place feet several inches apart and point them straight ahead. Place towel on floor in front of feet.

Steps of Exercise:

Step 1. Place toes on a towel near the middle. Your heels should be two inches above towel.

Step 2. Pull towel toward you by grasping towel with toes and curling toes under. Feet should not move.

Step 3. Continue bringing towel toward you until it is bunched in front of feet.

Repetitions: Do a minimum of six times, twice daily.

Comments: The patient can do towel tug-of-war if there are two people exercising.

F. Towel Turn

Starting position: Sit in chair with feet four inches apart and place flat on the edges of a towel.

Steps of exercise:

Step 1. Grasp the towel with the toes.

Step 2. While holding towel with toes, bring feet inward until they are facing each other.

Step 3. Relax toes to release towel. Return feet to starting position.

Step 4. Grasp towel with toes again and bring feet inward. The towel should be starting to be bunched between feet.

Step 5. Repeat exercise until the towel is bunched between feet.

Repetitions: Do a minimum of six times, twice daily.

9. Unless you suffer from a disease that requires that you remain sedentary, it is important in general to stay active. Walking is a wonderful way to exercise your feet. It not only improves your foot and leg circulation, but is also crucial for your general physical and mental health. If you have been sedentary or inactive for a long period of time, you must consult your physician before exercising.

10. Excessive weight is unhealthy for anyone at any age. Additional weight puts a tremendous strain on your feet and legs and every effort should be made to reduce and get down to the appropriate weight for your height and age. Many general health (as well as foot and leg) disorders can be prevented. Certainly the discomfort can be diminished by shedding unnecessary pounds.

11. Eight out of ten Americans suffer from some sort of foot and leg disorder. Many of these people assume that nothing can be done about it, that it is normal to have chronic foot and leg pain, lower backaches and fatigue, especially as they age.

This is simply not true and you should not accept this attitude. If you have no serious systematic diseases that could cause foot, leg, and lower back problems, then in addition to the regular exercises already mentioned, you should evaluate your foot and leg structure. Often, making an inlay to help compensate for abnormal foot and leg structure will help alleviate a lot of the skeletal symptoms described above. For a full understanding of this concept and what to do about it see appendix B—Foot Structure and Function and appendix D—Shoe Inserts You Can Make.

12. More specific and aggressive exercises for specific foot and leg problems can also be helpful. Obviously, if you have lead a sedentary existence, or you are being treated for something that you feel may interfere with these exercises, please consult your physician before starting.

A. For chronic pain and fatigue in the arches, the following simple exercises can be done daily:

- Sock-Gripping

Starting position: Sit with back straight in chair.

Bend legs to right angle. Place feet shoulder-width apart and point them straight ahead. Place a sock on the floor between feet.

Steps of exercise:

Step 1. Curl toes under as much as possible and grip sock firmly.

Step 2. Pivot on heels and move feet outward to stretch sock between feet.

Step 3. Remain on heels in outward position and lift sole of foot away from ground.

Step 4. Remain in this position and pull sock between feet as hard as possible for five seconds.

Step 5. Return to starting position. Repeat.

Repetitions: Do a minimum of six times, twice daily.

Comments: Do not move knees during exercise.

- Toe Rises

Starting position: Stand twelve inches away from and facing wall with back straight. Feet are eight to twelve inches apart, pointed out and flat on floor.

Steps of exercise:

Step 1. Rise on toes as high as possible.

Step 2. Hold position for five seconds. Repeat.

Repetitions: Do a minimum of ten times, twice daily.

B. For leg cramps here is a good ten-minute exercise routine for use both before and after athletic activity.

1. Wall-pushes with the knees bent, 30 seconds for each leg, twice. In this exercise keep your feet flat on the ground (don't lift the heel), with your weight on both legs. Repeat with the knees straight.

2. Toe-touches, 30 to 60 seconds each side (left leg crossed over right knee, then vice versa), twice. Go down slowly and do not bounce. Do not twist yourself that last inch in order to "touch" your toes momentarily; it will only make you tighter—and could cause injury. The only good stretch is one you can hold comfortably for 30 seconds.

- Assisted Leg Raise

Starting position: Lie flat on back with legs straight. Put belt or towel around left foot, holding ends.

Steps of exercise:

Step 1. Keep right leg on floor. Gently pull belt to raise left leg.

Step 2. Continue pulling belt until stretch discomfort is felt. Hold five seconds. Repeat.

Repetitions: Do a minimum of ten times for each leg, twice daily.

Comments: Do not force leg, pull belt only until stretch pain is felt.

3. Move your foot straight up (without lifting the leg) for a count of five, and relax. Repeat five times. The same exercise should be repeated with the foot turned inwards.

4. For lower back fatigue and aches: To further stretch the back, hold the left leg just below the knee and pull it toward your chest. Stretch and relax. Keep the back of your head down and then slowly curl your head up toward your bent knee. Repeat with other leg.

13. A simple way to help keep your feet and legs in shape and feeling good at the end of the day (or whenever they feel tired), is to elevate your feet and legs and move your toes up and down for about a minute. Rest for a minute or two and repeat up to ten times. For this exercise elevate your feet and legs while sitting or lying flat or sitting with your feet extended in front of you and elevated on two pillows. This should not be done if you have any history of blood clots or poor circulation. You should consult your physician ahead of time.

14. Avoid standing in one position for very long periods of time—it slows down the circulation. Take breaks and sit down or use high stools for chores or work that you must do for long periods. After resting, do #12 and #13 listed previously.

15. Many older people experience discomfort after walking and standing for long periods on the balls of their feet. Often the fat pad cushioning is no longer present, hence they are literally standing on bone. If this is the case, make an inlay to help cushion this part of your foot. (See appendix D, "Shoe inserts you can make" and also chapter 8, "Callouses.")

16. Massage is very helpful to alleviate normal aches and cramps from fatigue. (See chapter 24, "Cramps.")

17. Your feet are an integral part of your body. What happens to them usually has residual effects on the rest of the body. What happens to the body often shows up first in the feet.

Symptoms of Disease

Many serious systemic problems are associated with the aging process. These can affect the feet as primary problems, or produce the initial signs and symptoms of problems in other parts of the body. Some such conditions are arthritis, diabetes, various circulatory disorders, kidney disease, bone conditions, and lower back problems. If you notice any of the following symptoms you should make note of them and consult your podiatrist or physician for further evaluation.

- Cramps in the feet and legs at night.
- Numbness in the feet and legs at night.
- Cold feet.
- Feet that are always painful when walking.

1. If some of these symptoms go away after massaging the feet and legs, getting up and walking around, or dangling the feet over the edge of the bed, then these are sure signs that you may have a problem with circulation.

• Intermittent claudication is limping due to pain in the calves or back of the legs that only occurs with walking. It goes away when you sit down and rest. When this pain continues to occur but over shorter and shorter distances, you should be concerned.

• Brittleness of the toenails

• Lack of hair growth or normal hair growth.

• Shiny or waxy looking skin.

• Excessive swelling in the feet and ankles.

2. If you do have circulatory problems and cold feet, properly fitting support hose can be helpful. Also, sleep with wool socks at night and elevate room temperature. Do not use hot water bottles or heating pads in bed because they can be dangerous.

3. Anyone who has serious circulatory diseases should read over and carefully follow chapter 31, "Foot Care for the Diabetic."

4. If you suffer from foot problems like corns, callouses, bunions, hammertoes, etc., and have been told by doctors that you must live with them, or that the cure is worse than the problem, first try reading the appropriate chapter in the beginning of this book. If your self-help attempts fail, visit a good podiatrist. Improved, modern techniques can give most people permanent relief from many foot conditions. An older person in fairly good general health can reap as many benefits of prolonged relief as younger people can.

Chapter 31

Foot Care for the Diabetic

Diabetes is a disease in which the body cannot properly utilize its sugar intake. The sugar level builds up in the blood system and causes many negative changes. Diabetics are often more susceptible to infection, have problems in healing, and circulatory disorders, especially in the feet. Diabetics also have loss of sensitivity in the feet and thus ulcers, infections, and injury may be present without their knowledge.

It is thus extremely important for people who have diabetes to give special care to their feet. The idea is to avoid rather than to invite trouble that can lead to more serious problems including gangrene, loss of toe or toes, and in some cases, loss of life.

The following are important recommendations for the foot care of diabetics. All are necessary.

1. Clean your feet daily by bathing them in warm water and drying them carefully. Be sure to dry thoroughly between the toes. Do not use any rubbing action whatever on your feet and do not use very hot or very cold water.

2. Use a moisturizing cream on your feet both in the morning and at bedtime. For example, you can use a vegetable shortening or fifty-percent mixture of liquid Crisco oil and VASELINE,™ vitamin A cream, cocoa butter, a good body cream or similar emollients.

3. Inspect your feet carefully every day (tops, bottoms, and between your toes). Make sure you have no infection, redness, heat, swelling, pain, openings or ulcers, cuts or opened areas. If you note any of these signs or anything unusual, consult your podiatrist immediately.

4. You should not treat your own feet. If you have corns, callouses, nail problems, etc., the home care remedies suggested throughout this book are not for you. Periodic preventative visits to your podiatrist are strongly advised. These visits usually average from every three weeks to two months at most. The length of time between visits depends on you, the severity of your diabetes, and what your podiatrist recommends.

5. We do not even recommend that you cut your own toenails. However, if you insist, make sure that any instruments you use are clean. Wash them in soap and water and rinse off with

alcohol or any recognized antiseptic. Make sure all of the materials and suggested medications are clean and up-to-date. Put two tablespoons of mild household detergent into one and one-half gallons of warm water. Dip your feet into the water and soak for ten minutes. Dry your feet thoroughly and gently, especially between the toes. Apply an antiseptic solution or spray to the toenails. Trim and cut the toenails straight across. Always leave them a little longer than you think they should be cut. **ABSOLUTELY DO NOT ATTEMPT TO CUT INTO THE CORNERS—OR DIG UNDER THE NAIL OR CUTICLE—NO MATTER WHAT!**

If you are in pain because of this, see a podiatrist immediately. After you have finished cutting your nails, rinse the toes off with warm soap and water. Dry your feet thoroughly and gently especially between the toes. Apply an antiseptic liquid or spray.

6. **Caution: We do not recommend doing the above, but we know it is being done all the time and so we prefer that at least some professional guidance be given. Remember however: we do not condone this practice.**

7. Most self-treatment for corns, callouses, hammertoes, warts, etc., are not recommended. See a podiatrist.

Similarly, any cuts, cracks, sores, abrasions, and any other injuries should be treated only by a podiatrist. If you do sustain such an injury, attend to it immediately and call your doctor. When attending to it, do the following:

A. Wash the area carefully with soap and water.

B. Make sure to remove all foreign material.

C. Apply an antiseptic.

D. Cover with a sterile 2 × 2 gauze pad and non-allergic paper tape.

E. Call your podiatrist.

8. Never use over-the-counter medications such as commercial or corn remedies unless prescribed by your podiatrist. This can cause serious problems even in people with healthy feet.

9. If you have a problem with excessive foot perspiration, you might first try using a mild talcum powder on your feet and in your socks. However, if the problem still occurs, see chapter 13, "Sweaty and Smelly Feet" or seek professional care.

10. If for any reason you see the need to use tape on your feet, (without your podiatrist's knowledge), do not use so-called regular adhesive-backed tape. Use the non-allergic tapes that peel away from the skin easily and are less abrasive to your skin tissue.

Shoe Do's and Don'ts

1. Be careful in choosing shoe wear. (See appendix C—Shoes.) Dress shoes should have soft leather uppers. Athletic shoes should have soft nylon uppers. Both these types of shoes are less likely to irritate your feet, probably will conform easily to any lumps or bumps, and will allow your feet to breathe appropriately.

A. Shoes made of artificial upper material are not porous and are usually too stiff for proper comfort.

B. Shoes must fit properly. They should not feel tight.

C. Change shoes daily to allow them to dry out.

D. Feet normally swell in the course of the day. Thus, it's best to shop for new shoes when feet are at their largest size—in the evenings. Be careful when buying high boots. Women's boot styles are especially likely to constrict the lower leg circulation of even people with healthy circulation. Diabetics should avoid these boots.

Hosiery Do's and Don'ts

1. Wear properly fitted socks.
2. Do not wear tube socks that are supposedly made to fit several foot sizes.
3. Do not wear socks with tight-elastic top bands.
4. Do not wear non-prescribed support hose because they may be too constrictive.
5. The best socks are wool, cotton, or nylon-blend socks.
6. Socks should be clean and changed every day.
7. Do not wear hosiery that needs to be mended. The mending will often lead to the formation of seams that can be irritating.
8. Do not wear anything tight around the legs or ankles that might interfere with the circulation to your feet.
9. Don't wear restrictive circular-shaped fibers.

Appendix A

All About Podiatrists

1. Definition:

"Podiatry is that profession of the health sciences which deals with the examination, diagnosis, treatment, and prevention of diseases, conditions, and malfunctions affecting the human foot and its related or governing structures, by employment of medical, surgical or other means." *—Adopted by American Podiatry Association House of Delegates.*

2. Education:

The pre-requisites for admission and criteria used in the admissions process by schools of podiatric medicine are identical to those of the traditional medical schools. A minimum of three years of pre-medical study at an accredited college or university, and a satisfactory score on the New-Medical College Admissions Test (New-MCAT). Better than 90% of those students entering a school of podiatry have Baccalaureate Degrees or higher, prior to the admission to the four year course in a college of podiatric medicine.

3. Colleges:

There are seven colleges of podiatric medicine in the United States. They are located in New York City, Philadelphia, Cleveland, Chicago, San Francisco, Des Moines, Iowa, and Miami Shores, Florida.

4. Curriculum:

The curriculum at the colleges of podiatric medicine is, in effect, a "single tract" medical education with special emphasis on the lower extremity, but provides a general medical curriculum parallel to that of traditional medical schools. Curricula offered by the individual colleges consist of more than 4,000 hours of instruction distributed throughout four academic years. Curricula in the first two years are predominantly in the basic sciences, and the final two years concentrate on clinical training and practice. Required courses include anatomy, physiology, biochemistry, pharmacology, microbiology, pathology, general and podiatric surgery and general and podiatric medicine, in addition to specific courses which relate to clinical practice. All the colleges confer the degree Doctor of Podiatric Medicine (DPM). During the last two years of the educational program, the student spends a major portion of his time in the study of podiatric medicine and surgery and its relation to the general health, well being and emergency care of patients. This study is accomplished in the clinics of the colleges, their allied clinical programs, affiliated teaching hospitals, long term care facilities, and private offices.

5. Podiatric Residency:

Over 50% of the graduates from the colleges of podiatric medicine enter post-graduate residency training programs of one, two or three years' duration. Such programs are carried out in teaching hospitals. The resident receives additional training in podiatric medicine and surgery and serves in rotation and emergency services, anesthesiology, radiology, general medicine, pathology, general surgery, and podiatric surgery. Programs also include experience in other services such as pediatrics, dermatology, neurology, orthopedics, and physical medicine and rehabilitation. Both the professional and post-graduate education programs stress an awareness of the vital need to promote cooperative relationships between podiatry and the other primary health professions in the appropriate delivery of quality health care services.

6. Licensing

Podiatrists are licensed in all 50 states to treat the foot medically, mechanically and surgically. Foot and leg problems seen on an everyday basis by podiatrists include:

A. Infants and children
   1. Foot deformities requiring correction through bracing, casting or surgery.
   2. Flat feet
   3. Pidgeon toeing
   4. Outtoeing
   5. Leg cramps
   6. Skin conditions

B. Injury
   1. Fractures and dislocations
   2. Sprains and strains
   3. Lacerations, cuts and bruises
   4. Foreign bodies; splinters, glass, stings
   5. Burns

C. Skin conditions
   1. Fungus infection (athletes foot)
   2. Allergies
   3. Nail disease
   4. Corns and callouses
   5. Plantar warts
   6. Skin tumors
   7. Foot odor and excessive sweating
   8. Blisters

D. Sports medicine
   1. Prevention of athletic injuries
   2. Treatment of athletic injuries

E. Bone and joint problems
   1. Bunions
   2. Arthritis
   3. Heel spurs
   4. Hammertoes
   5. Arch problems

F. Aged
   1. Diabetic foot problems
   2. Circulatory problems

Appendix B

Foot Structure and Function

The foot has two basic functions. One is to adapt to the surfaces on which we walk or run, and absorb the shock of impact; and the other is to accept the body weight from above and move it forward.

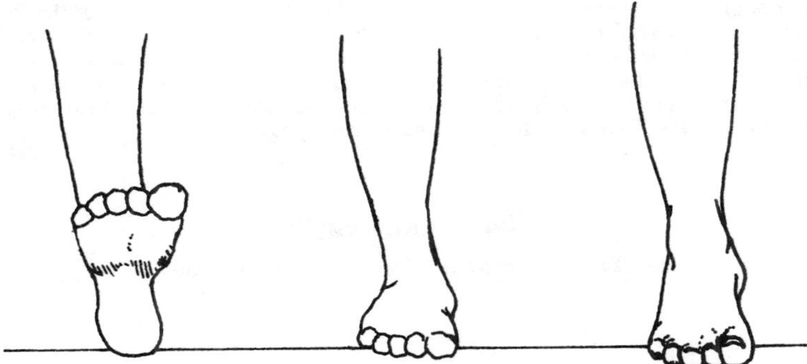

When the "normal" foot strikes the ground, it contacts on the outside of the heel and then rolls inward and downward and the arch lowers a little. This series of motions is called *pronation*. It allows the foot to become loose and mobile in order to be an effective adapter and shock absorber. After the foot has landed firmly, and is bearing the full weight of the body, the directions of the foot movements reverse. The arch starts to rise, and the foot starts to roll upwards and outwards, becoming very rigid and stable in order to lift the weight of the body and move it forward. This series of movements is called *supination*.

In order to accomplish these movements, the joints and muscles of the entire lower extremity, from the ankle to the hip, go through a special sequence of motions. The timing is extremely important. If the foot goes from pronation to supination smoothly and on time, no strain or loss of efficient motion occurs. However, if it pronates excessively, the weight of the body falls on the foot at the wrong time. Instead of being a rigid, stable structure, the foot is a "loose bag of bones" and cannot possibly propel the body forward efficiently. Instead of being in a strong supinated position, it is in a pronated or weakened state. This is the cause of many overuse injuries in athletics. It also explains why people who pronate excessively may have their performance adversely affected. Muscles which are designed for stabilization are called upon to help propel; and propeller muscles are forced to help with the stabilization. When the various muscle groups of the lower extremities are called upon to do work that they were not intended to do, they become strained and performance levels are diminished. Another problem with excessive pronation is that body weight is thrust on the foot at a time when it is unstable. The bones are subjected to abnormal stresses, which can lead to stress fractures, bone spur formations, enlargements of bones called exostoses, joint injuries, bursitis, and arthritis. And, with the muscles forced to do the wrong work, as described above, stresses are created which can lead to muscle and tendon injuries. In some cases, excessive stresses are transmitted through the legs to the skeletal structure above, producing many of the knee, hip, and lower back injuries seen in runners. Because of evolutionary failures, most of us—something like 80 to 90 percent of us—have feet which are sufficiently imperfect in structure to cause them to function defectively to some extent.

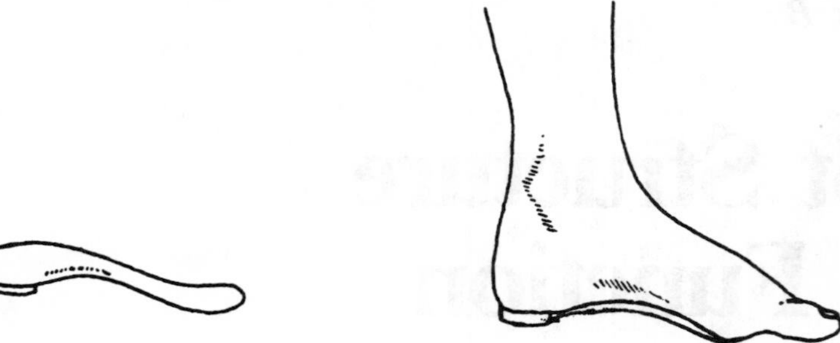

Each one of us is born with a particular structural relationship between the front of the foot, back of the foot, leg, and supporting surface. This is known as the neutral position. This position is neither "normal" or "abnormal," but is the one an individual must function with. If a person's neutral position is such that he or she strikes the ground at heel contact excessively to the outside of the heel or front of the foot (forefoot), then it is obvious that this foot must pronate excessively or abnormally in order to get the inside of the foot to contact the ground. To alleviate this problem, an orthotic device can be made which eliminates abnormal pronation and allows the foot and leg to function with maximum efficiency. An orthotic is a scientifically fabricated device which is contoured to fit each individual foot and may have rearfoot and forefoot posts which represent specific degrees of biomechanical correction in order to retain a proper relationship between the forefoot, rearfoot, and leg, and the supporting surface. To have such a device made, see a podiatrist.

Self Examination

Stand in front of a mirror nude, or have someone directly observe your structure.

1. *From the front:*

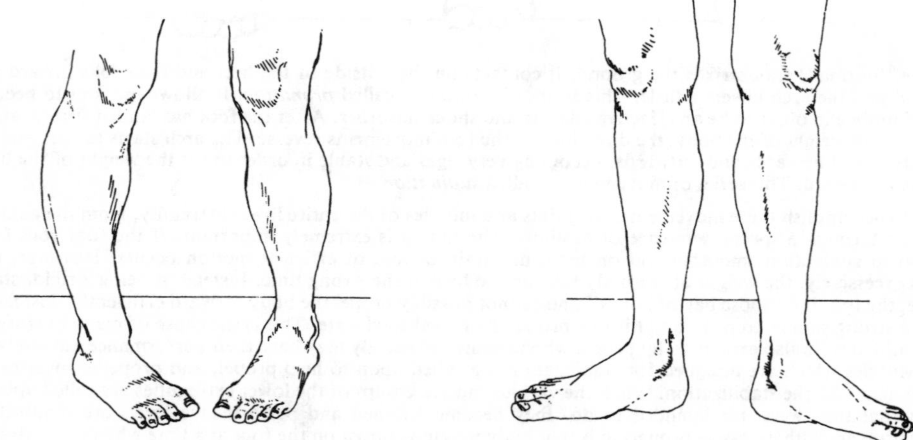

► Do your toes turn in, toward each other (toe in; pigeon-toed)?
► Do your toes turn out, away from each other (toe-out; duck-walk)?

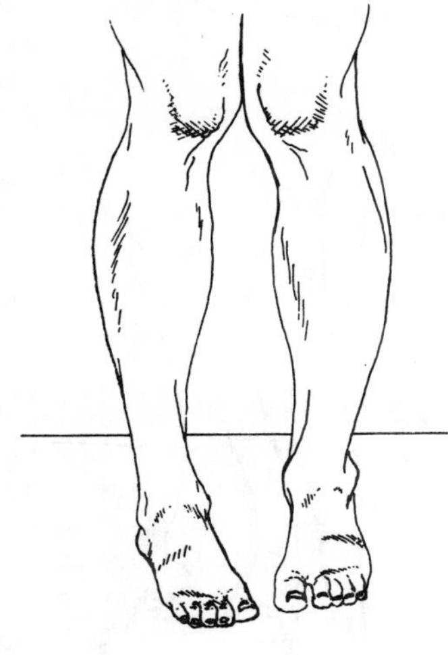

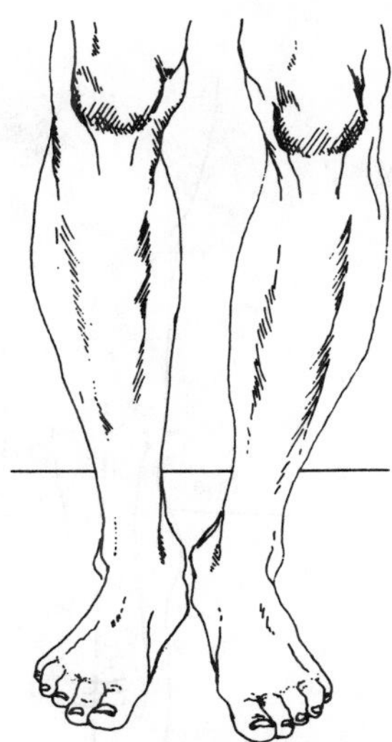

► When your legs are together, do your knees touch, and is there a space between your ankles (knock-knees)?
► When your legs are together, do your ankles touch, and is there a space between your knees (bow-legs)?

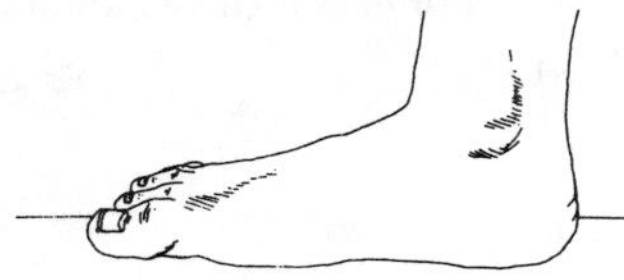

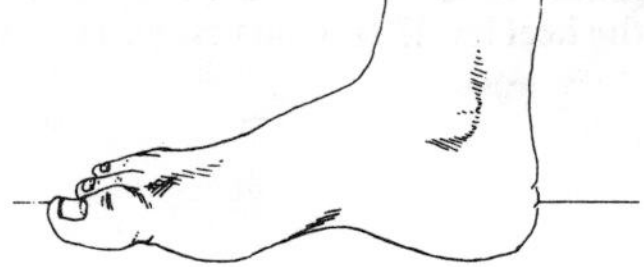

► Are your feet flat?
► Are your arches high?

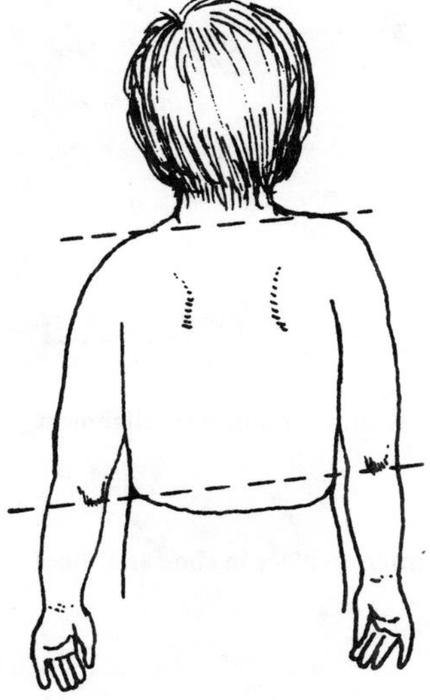

► Is one shoulder lower?
► Is one arm longer?
► Is one hip higher?

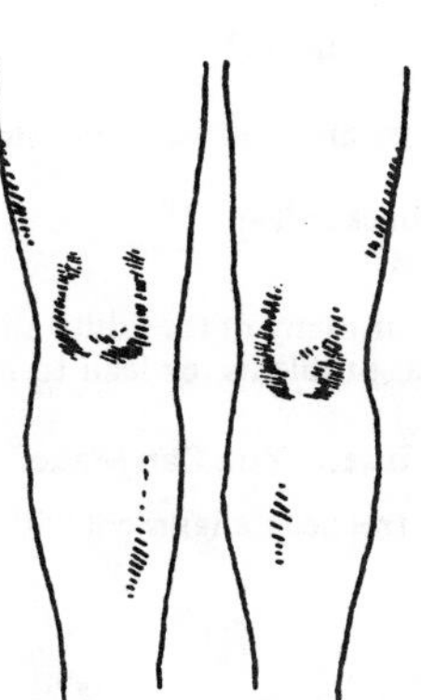

► Is one knee cap higher?

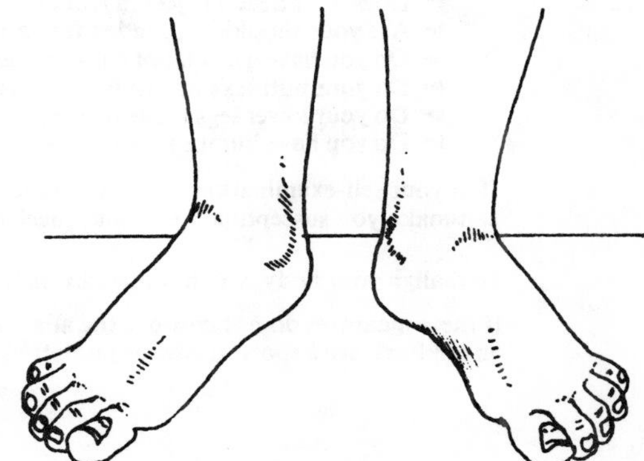

► Is one foot flat while the other has a high arch?

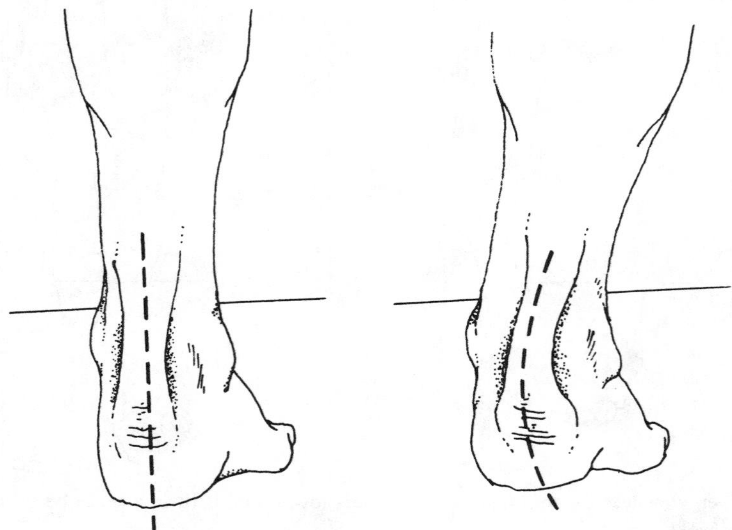

3. *From the back:*
   ► Does the achilles tendon look straight up and down at the back of the leg . . . or does it curve outward when it gets to the heel level? If it curves, you probably pronate excessively.

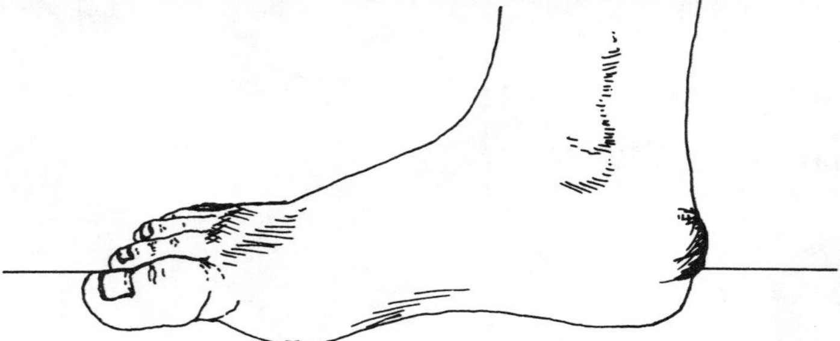

4. *From the side:*
   ► Does your head project in front of your shoulders?
   ► Are your shoulders rounded forward?
   ► Do you have a small pot belly that exercise and diet won't take away?
   ► Do your buttocks protrude excessively?
   ► Do your lower legs curve from front to back?
   ► Do you have bumps in back of your heels?

If in your self-examination you have found one or many of the faulty alignments listed, your improper alignment can make you susceptible to various mechanical problems, or lead to injury.

To realign your body, see the appendix on Shoe Inserts You Can Make.

If these measures do not improve the alignment (recheck alignment with proper insert in place in shoe and shoes on the feet), see a sports medicine podiatrist.

Appendix C

Shoes

Shoes should be made to accommodate not only the shape of the foot, but the function of the foot as it helps the body to move. Since the feet function quite differently with different kinds of activity, this appendix is divided into four sections—walking shoes and questions of a general nature, shoes for babies, shoes for older children, and running shoes.

Walking Shoes And General Information

1. What should you look for in trying on a new pair?

Consumers are often advised to buy shoes at the end of the day, when their feet are more likely to be tired and swollen. Feet begin to swell as soon as you take your first steps after arising in the morning. If you cannot shop at the end of the day, at least walk around a bit before going to the store. This way you'll be assured of a better fit.

Buy shoes at a store that *uses a Brannock device.* This is a foot-measuring device for determining exact shoe size. If the salesperson asks you your shoe size instead of measuring your foot, you may be in the wrong store. When you are being measured, stand on the foot being measured. Most people have a larger foot; generally the right foot is slightly larger than the left. Fit your shoes to the larger foot. How the shoe feels is just as important as what size it is. So don't decide that a particular shoe is for you unless it feels good.

Allow a half-inch between the tip of your shoes and your longest toe. A finger's width of extra space is about right.

Examine the shoe. Make sure it bends easily across the ball of the foot, that it is not concave between the arch and the heel, and that the shoe slips easily over the instep without "cutting" (you should be able to "pinch up" the leather across the ball). The heel should fit snugly and the shoe should not slip or rub anywhere. It should feel good the moment you try it on. It should not have to be "broken in."

Be wary of certain high-fashion shoe styles. The foot is squarish in shape—not pointy. Pointy-toed shoes do not provide sufficient room. Square, high toe-boxes are the best for your feet. A steel shank is also a good idea because it helps retain the shape of the shoe.

When you try shoes on, wear the same socks or stockings you expect to wear with them. Sweat socks with dress shoes won't tell you how the shoes will feel with light cotton socks.

For a good fit, your best bet could well be the small family or independent shoe store, although many of the larger chains are now striving to provide better service in fitting a pair of shoes.

"Professional shoe-fitters" will take the time to see that you get a proper fit. "Shoe salesmen" will try to sell you whatever they can. You'll find both types at your local shoe store. Shoe-fit is so important to your well-being that if you are not completely satisfied with your service ask for someone else or go to another store.

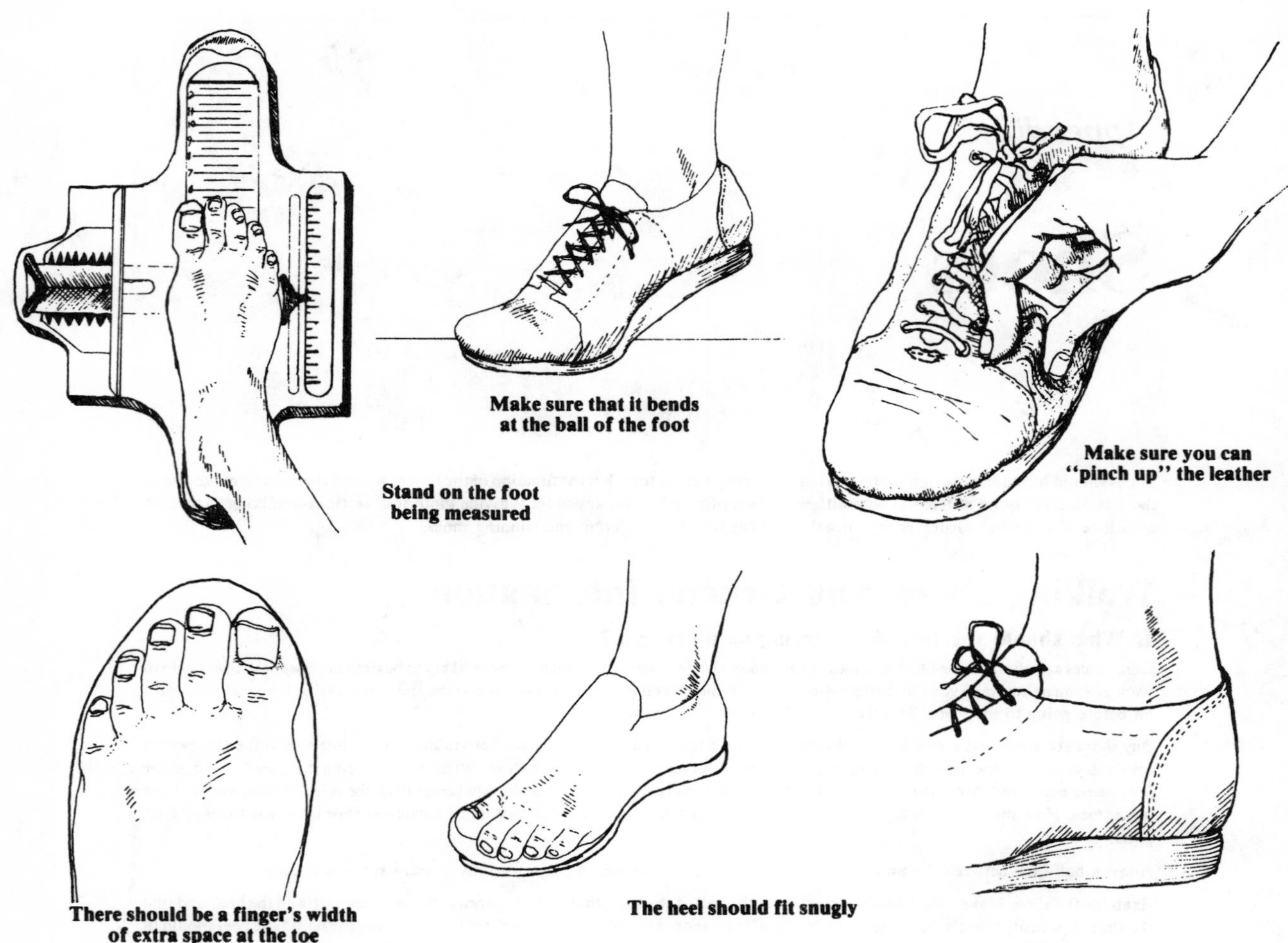

2. What Is The Best Material For Shoes To Be Made Of?

Buy leather shoes. They are more expensive, but leather has important features that make it superior to so-called man-made materials. It has some of the same properties as human skin. It is moldable and really adapts to the shape of the foot. Since your foot may change size and shape during the day, leather can accommodate it by stretching or contracting. When shoe leather "breathes," an exchange of moisture and absorption takes place. Leather is not only a superior absorber of moisture, it can vaporize this moisture into the air. This capability plays a key role in hygiene and comfort and discourages the buildup of bacteria within the shoe. If this vaporization does not occur, the feet get hot and perspire profusely; these conditions favor infection, odor, and athletes foot.

3. Do Shoes Cause Foot Problems?

Many people blame shoes for their foot problems, but the causes often lie elsewhere. If you have a deformity such as a bunion or a hammertoe, it's probable that you would have developed it whether you had worn shoes or not. Shoes, however, can certainly aggravate foot problems that already exist. And shoes—particularly athletic shoes—can protect the feet from shock, friction, and stress that might otherwise be intolerable.

Shoe design and materials play a role in foot problems, but so do heredity, hard surfaces, and other factors. A prominent podiatrist once said, "A pair of shoes will not make the feet well, any more than a new hat will cure a headache."

4. Rotate your shoes.

Never wear the same pair two days in a row as it takes 24 hours for a shoe to dry out after you have worn it. Remember that the fungus that causes Athlete's Foot infections thrives in damp, dark, warm places, and you can't find a better example of such a growth environment than the inside of a shoe.

It is even smart to rotate them during the day. If you are wearing stylish shoes that are not perfectly comfortable, or boots, for example, change sometime during the day to a more comfortable pair.

Wearing running shoes to and from work and changing to stylish shoes while at work has become very popular. It is not at all uncommon to see women in full executive business dress walking into their offices in a pair of "Nikes."

Give your feet a break during the day by kicking off your shoes while at your desk. Stretch them real good and rotate them at the ankles. Walking in socks on a carpet is also very relaxing. Try this when your fellow employees are not around.

These little tips can make your day much more pleasant. Remember, "A pretty face starts at your feet."

5. Do "orthopedic" or "corrective" shoes really help?

Unfortunately, there is no ready-made or even custom-made shoe that has a sound mechanism built into it to control the way we walk. Most authorities agree that "corrective" shoes do not correct. Rather, abnormal stresses put on the feet by unhealthy motion patterns will be directly transferred to the shoe itself and the shoe will then conform and break down.

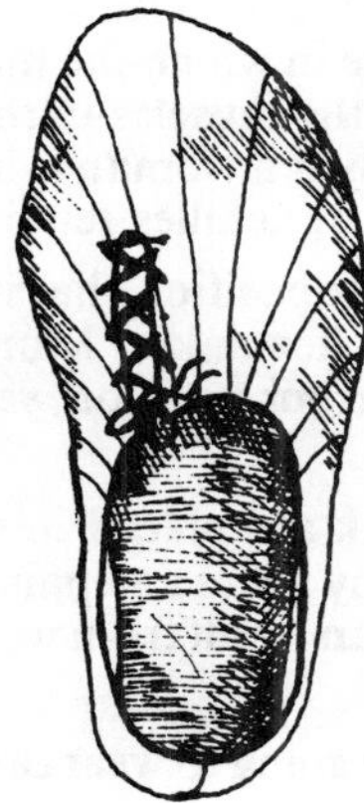

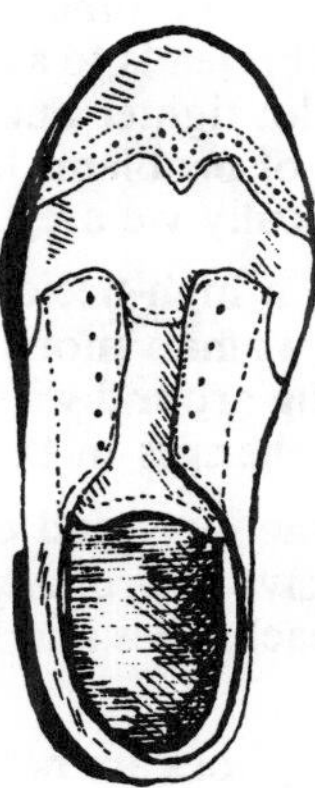

A word about children's orthopedic shoes. We have seen too many cases of children who have had a deformity at birth and were put into "corrective" shoes. Orthopedic shoes for children should be used only temporarily to retain a correction made by something else (casting or surgery), or in the mildest of foot deformities. Even in these cases, the shoe will only work until the abnormal forces and stresses placed upon it break it down. These shoes are so stiff that the amount of force it takes to bend the sole may actually be more than the child weighs. Because of this lack of flexibility, such shoes actually cause more foot problems than they prevent.

High-Heeled Shoes

High-heeled shoes are any shoes with heel heighths over an inch and one-half. Although many women wear them as high as three and four inches, the reality is that high-heeled shoes are not good for anyone's feet. Yet because of sexual and status ramifications, the high-heeled shoe probably will never go out of existence.

1. Here are some of the problems that high heels can cause.

   A. The weight distribution of your body normally should be about forty percent on the front of the foot and sixty percent in the heel. In high-heeled shoes, eighty percent of the body weight is thrust forward—the higher the heel the higher the percentage of weight. In addition, your foot is usually squeezed into very narrow-toed shoes. Obviously, many foot problems such as hammertoes, bunions, corns, and calluses, which may have been dormant and thus not a problem, will be exacerbated by wearing these shoes.

   B. It is important to note that these problems are not caused by these shoes but that irritation from the shoes can aggravate existing problems.

   C. The calf muscles become shorter if a woman wears high-heeled shoes for a prolonged period of time. This leads to a drastic muscle imbalance in which the muscles in the back of the legs are a lot tighter and more contracted than the muscles in the front. This can lead to a myriad of problems in the lower leg especially if a woman is involved in fitness activities. Specifically we are talking about shin splints, achilles tendinitis, etc.

   D. The ankle in a high-heeled shoe is placed in such a position that it's in a weakened state, making a woman more susceptible to twisting her ankle. Moreover, the subtle trauma of walking around with the ankle in this precarious position, year after year, can lead to arthritic changes in the ankle joint.

   E. The knees, the hips, and especially the lower back are placed in positions that are really not conducive to proper posture. Therefore, many aches and pains in the knees and hips, especially backaches and lower back problems, can result from wearing high-heeled shoes.

2. Since high-heeled shoes are here to stay and women are going to wear them, here are some recommendations that may be helpful.

   A. If you do wear high-heeled shoes (two-, three- or four-inch heels), then we suggest you rotate them during the week. For example, one day wear a three-inch heel; the next day wear a two and one-half; and the next a two-inch heel, etc.

   B. You may also change shoes and heel heighths during a particular day.

   C. We recommend that every woman own a pair of running or tennis shoes that are fairly flat and have rounded toes. These shoes should be worn at nights and on weekends.

   D. In addition to that we recommend calf-stretching exercises.

   E. Flat shoes with rounded toes are probably the best shoes the day after you wear high-heeled shoes at night. This change in heel height will help stretch the achilles tendon out. The tightness of the achilles tendon or calf muscle complex and hamstring muscles in the back of the leg and thigh often leads to lower back problems and problems with other parts of the skeletal system.

Appendix D

Shoe Inserts You Can Make

This section contains instructions for making inserts (1) to balance your foot to relieve corns and callouses; (2) to provide a temporary orthotic-type device or varus wedge; or (3) to compensate for a difference in length between your two legs. The conditions under which each of these adjustments may be called for are described in the chapters on specific types of foot conditions.

Materials:

1. A pair of your shoes
2. Graph paper (10" x 12")
3. Lipstick
4. Two 4" x 8" squares of adhesive foam
5. 1/8" adhesive foam
6. Piece of calf or kidskin leather
7. Spenco inlay or other store bought inlay as an alternative

Caution: Minor muscle aches in the legs, hips, feet or back are normal during the break-in phase for these inserts. Wear them for one hour the first day, adding on an hour each day until you can wear them comfortably all day long. Once you can wear them comfortably walking for six to eight hours straight or more, you can use them for athletic activity. If unusual discomfort develops, see a podiatrist.

Note: Unless you have one leg longer than another, whatever you make to put under one foot or in one shoe, you should do for the other.

1. To balance your foot . . .

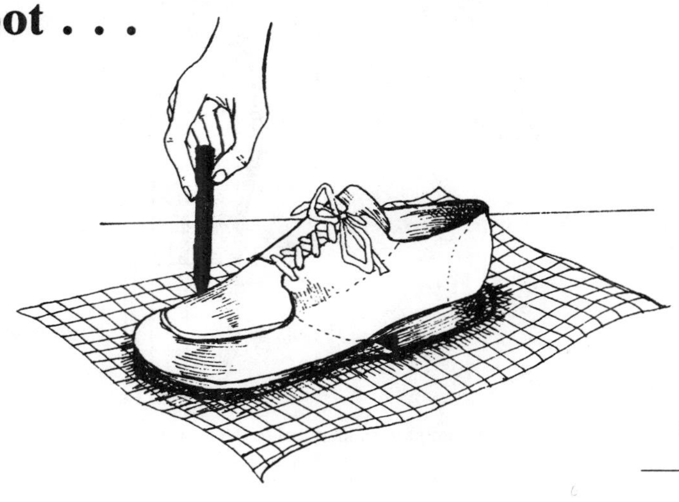

1. Place your shoe on a sheet of paper (preferably graph paper) and trace its outline.

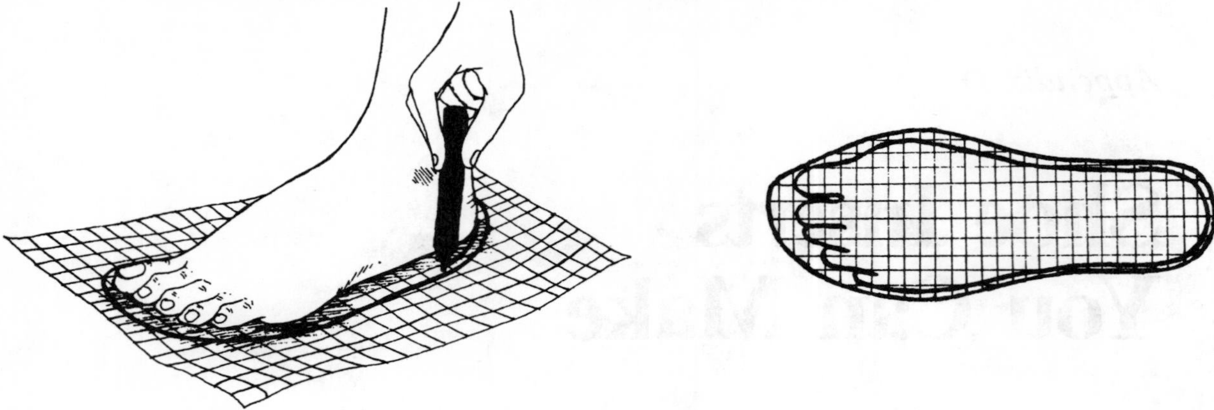

2. Step onto the shoe outline (center your bare foot in it) and trace the foot.

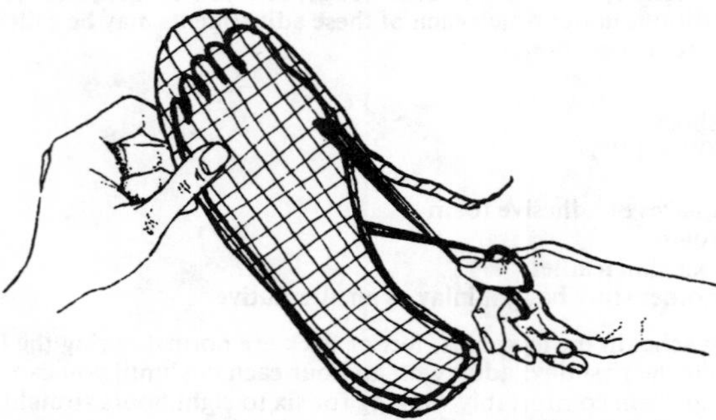

3. Cut out the foot pattern (it should end up about ¼" smaller all around than the shoe diagram). The pattern should fit inside the shoe.

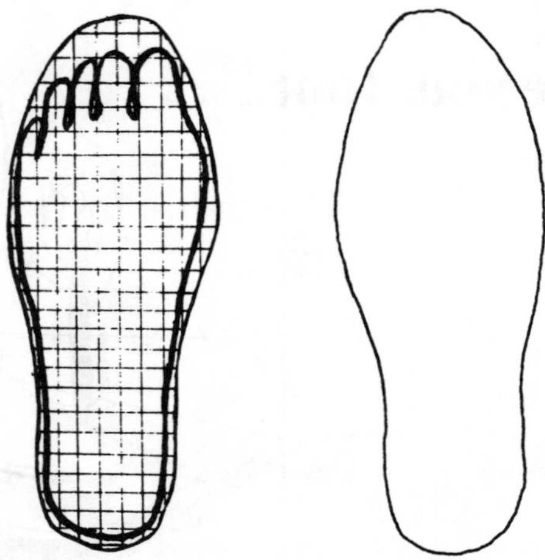

4. Cut a second pattern identical to the first, then turn it over for the other foot.

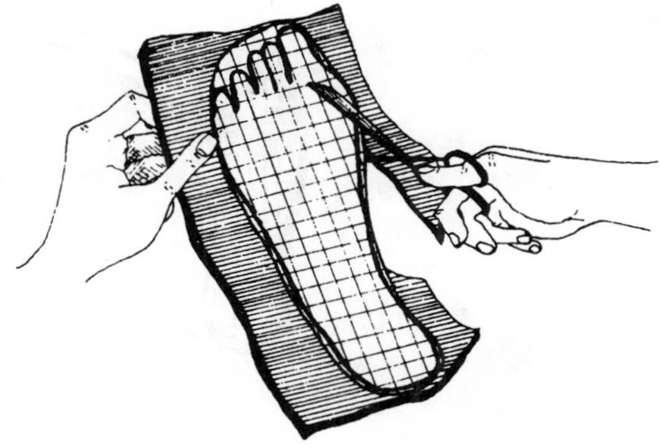

5. Tape each pattern onto kidskin leather and foam (leather on top) and cut out. (A full length, commercially available, innersole sized according to shoe size or a Spenco type insole may be substituted for the leather and foam that you are making from scratch. If you decide on this substitution then skip step six; and where it specifies kidskin and adhesive, use the store bought insert instead.
6. Attach the adhesive side of the foam to the underside of the piece of kidskin leather. If you don't have *adhesive* foam, you may glue the foam to the leather using rubber cement, barge cement or one of the new instant-stick glues.
7. Color the callouses on the bottom of the foot with lipstick.

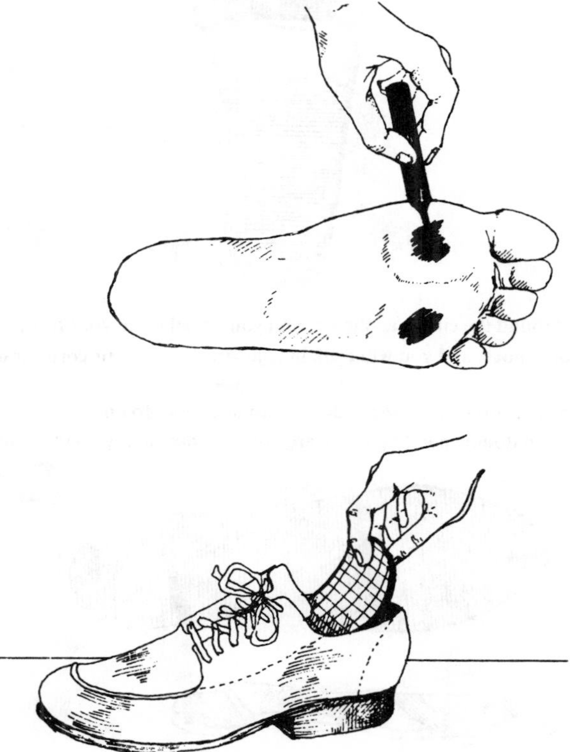

8. Put patterns into the shoes, then walk around for five minutes (do both feet at the same time).

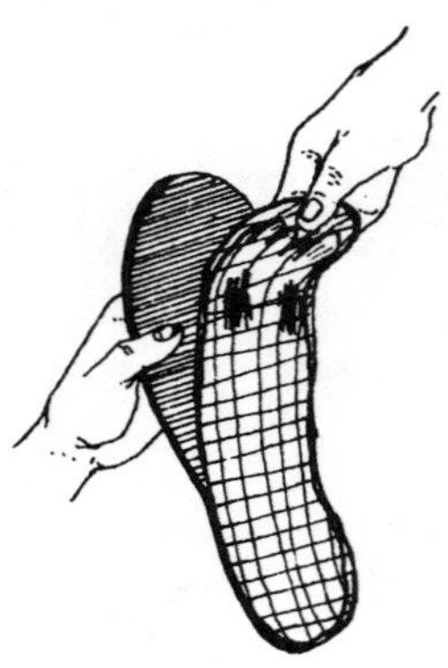

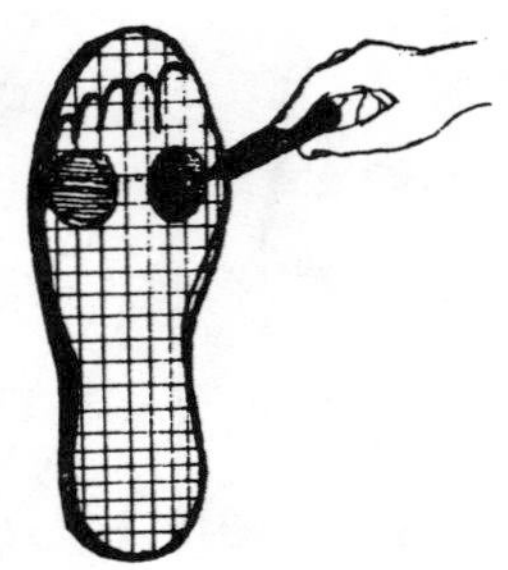

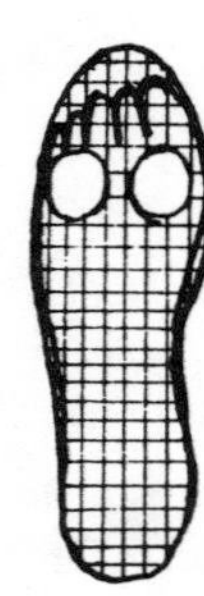

9. Remove the shoes and take the patterns out. Put circles around the lipstick marks on the pattern and cut out circles. Then tape the pattern onto the bottom (foam) side of the insole and color in the circles. Make sure you use the proper pattern for each foot.

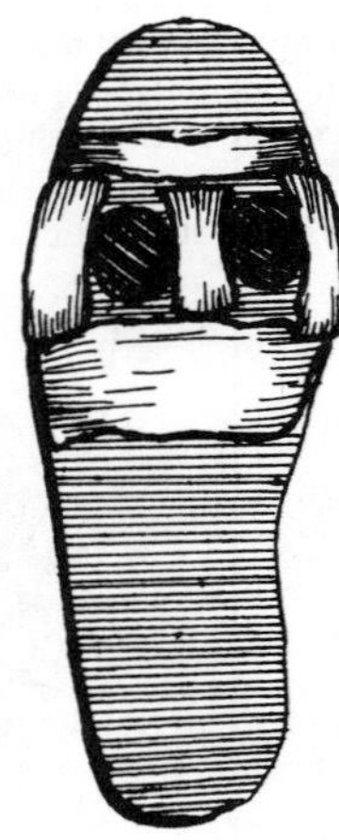

10. Place 1/8'' foam strips around the circles as shown, and you've balanced your foot.
11. Wear this inlay in all your shoes, and you will walk in comfort; in fact your corns or callouses in many cases may disappear altogether.
12. If you need more support, or if the insert wears down, just add more foam.
13. For additional support, add double padding in the arch or heel, depending on the pain.

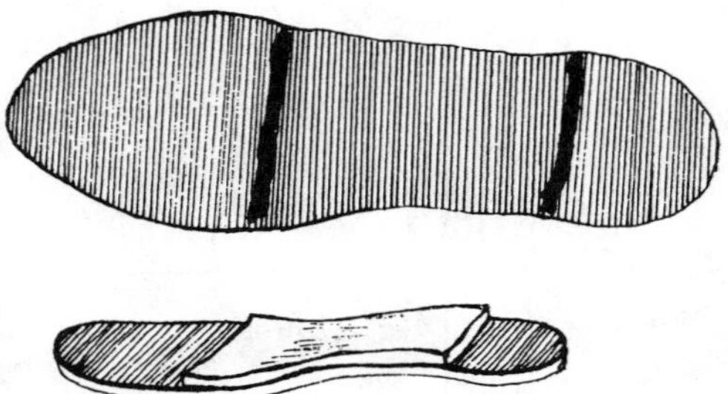

14. For heel pain or arch pain put a line of lipstick across the front of your heel, and another behind the ball of your foot. Step on the pattern in shoe as above. Fill the area between the two lines with a double thickness of 1/8'' foam.

2. To Make a Temporary Orthotic-type insert (varus wedge . . .)

1. Purchase a pair of Spenco inlays or make a full length leather and foam insert as described in steps one through six.
2. On the bottom of the inlay, mark the center of the heel (bisect lengthwise) with a pen.
3. Mark the widest portion (across the ball joint), bisecting the ball widthwise (extend from behind big toe to just behind little toe). Mark another line parallel and one inch behind the ball joint line (both of these lines will course slightly diagonally across the bottom of the inlay).

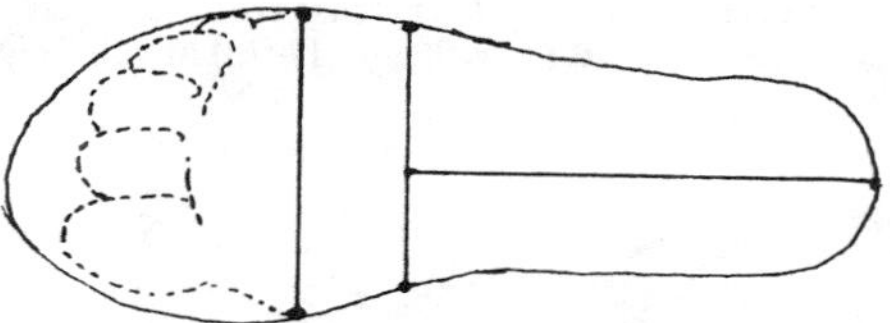

4. Bisect the second line, extend the heel bisection line until the two lines intersect.

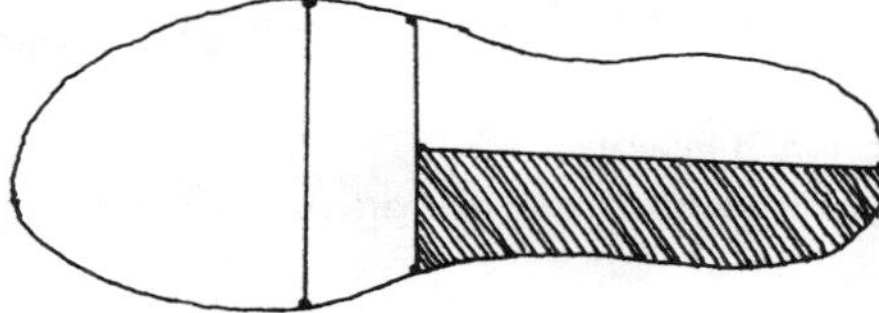

5. Fill the entire *inside* portion of the inlay between the lines with 1/8" to 1/4" adhesive foam or felt (if you don't have access to the adhesive, use glues previously discussed).
6. Bevel the edges of the foam or felt with scissors or file.
7. When this insert is placed into your shoe it will hold your foot in a varus position.

3. Heel Pads—Heel Lifts

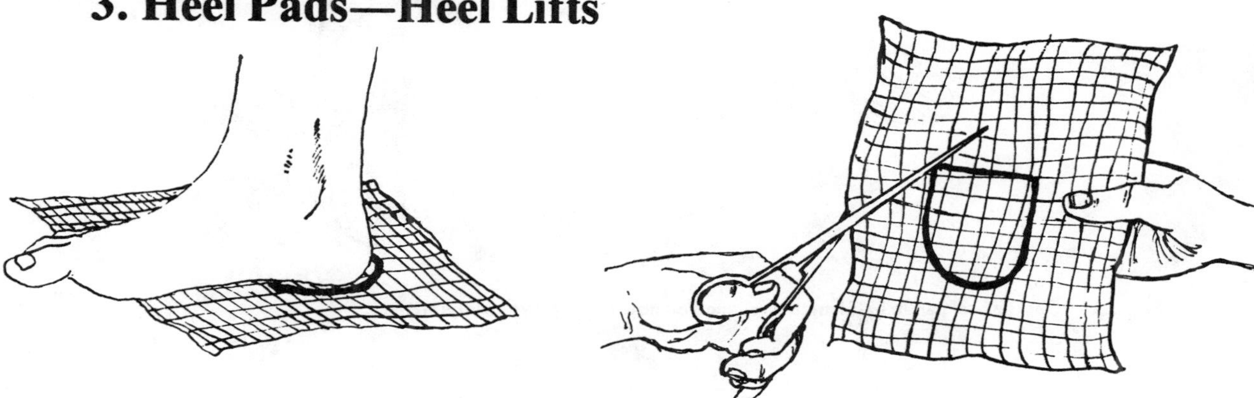

Trace the outer perimeter of the heel onto a piece of paper and cut out.

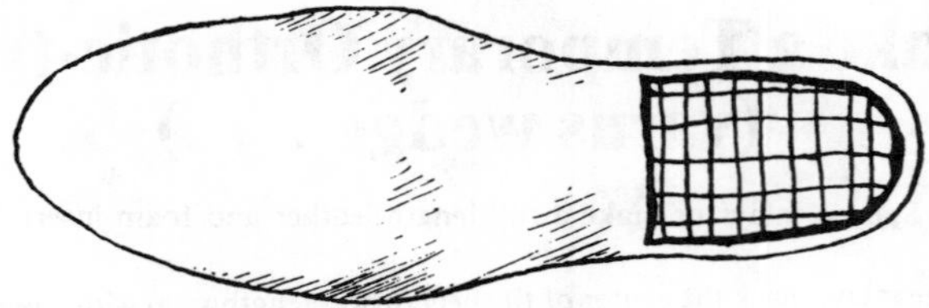

Trim the patterned shape of the heel all around so that your pattern now is ¼'' smaller than the heel of your shoe.

Take a piece of 1/8'' or 1/4'' felt (you may want to increase thickness later as needed) and tape the pattern onto it. Cut out the pattern and you will wind up with a heel lift that will fit into all of your shoes.

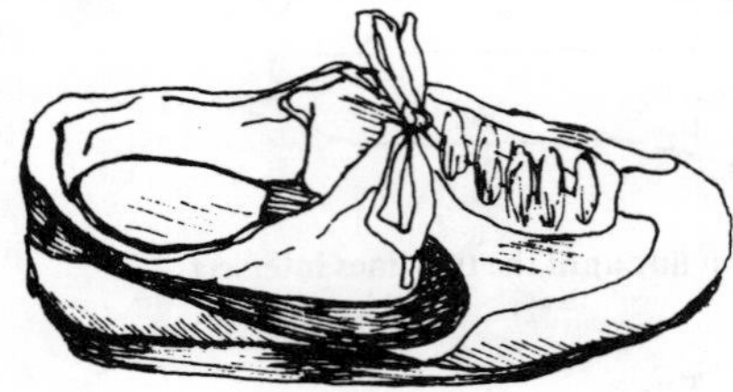

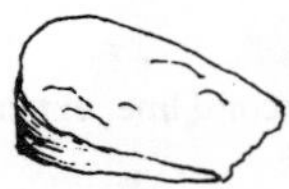

Thin down the lift toward the front if indicated.

For those conditions that require two lifts, place the pattern on the second piece of felt, cut out, and thin down the front as described.

4. Varus Heel Wedge

1. Repeat steps one through four in the heel pad section.
2. Place the completed heel pad on a flat surface right side up (sticky side down if adhesive).

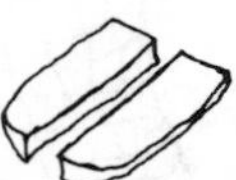

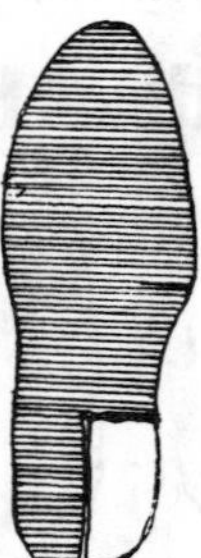

3. Cut the heel pad in half lengthwise, and you now have two varus heel wedges.

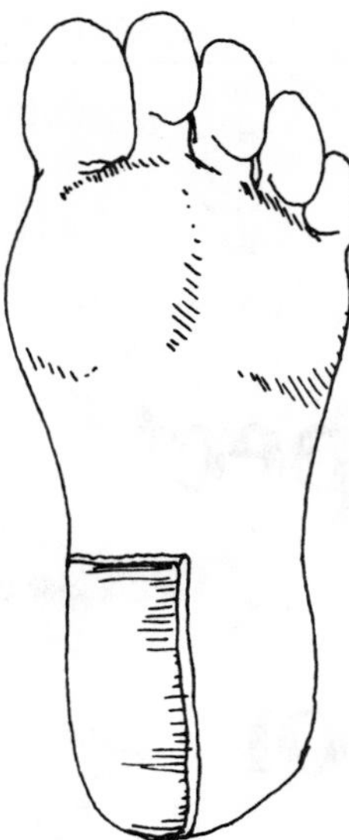

4. For placing the wedge directly onto your heel, or onto the bottom of an inlay, take the left half of the pad thin down the inner (straight) edge. Turn the pad upside down (sticky side up, if adhesive) and adhere to the inside of the bottom of the left heel.

5. Use the left half for the left heel.

6. For placing the wedge directly into your *right* shoe, take the *left* half of the pad and thin down the inner straight border. Place right side up (sticky side down if adhesive) into the inside of the shoe on the left side over the heel.

7. For placing the wedge directly into your left shoe, take the right half of the heel pad and follow step six above.

Appendix E

What to Expect When You Visit a Doctor

The Foot Doctor's Arsenal

Well, you've tried the foot doctoring yourself and you still have a problem. What's next?

1. The Right Doctor.

A. Fully 80 percent of the population will experience a foot problem during their lifetime. Options are available for treatment of feet. It no longer is okay to leave it up to the doctor. The consumer deserves the right to decide his fate. Your choice is a podiatrist or an orthopedist in most cases. Podiatrists are doctors of podiatric medicine. They treat diseases and injuries of the *foot and related structures* by medical, mechanical, and surgical means (see appendix A). Orthopedists are doctors of medicine. They treat diseases and injuries of *all bones and joints* by medical, mechanical and surgical means. No matter which one you choose, speak up loud and clear for yourself. A frank discussion of the risks and benefits of the treatment program the doctor outlines, as well as his or her qualifications for being able to provide it, is in order.

Ask such questions as, "What are my alternatives to this treatment that you have proposed, doctor?" "Are there less extensive, less painful, less disabling procedures available than the one you suggested?" "What can go wrong?" "How many of these procedures do you do each year, doctor?" *Remember,* just because a doctor has a license to perform a procedure on a foot doesn't mean he can do it well or can even make a proper judgment as to which procedure is the best approach to a particular problem. If my bunion has to be corrected, I want it done by a doctor who performs five bunion operations a week, not one who does one every three to six months.

It is also a good idea to be able to talk to other patients who have been to that doctor to see if the general scenario they were given prior to treatment was pretty much what occurred during and after it. If the doctor says that a patient can return to work in two days and he's still not back at work in six weeks, I want to know why before that doctor touches me.

Many patients are afraid to ask questions because they fear their doctor's reaction. Too often they then enter into foot treatment with unnecessary fears and anxieties stemming from a lack of knowledge about their problems. The principles of foot treatment are relatively simple, and a frank and careful explanation of what lies ahead, along with clear and sensible answers to the many questions patients wish to ask, can go a long way to minimize fears. This is particularly true when foot surgery is going to be performed.

Doctors are sometimes so busy that they tell the patient not to worry about what is coming (which may be very routine to them) and thus fail to fully explain details or adequately dispel fears. If the doctor is unwilling to explain in detail why the suggested treatment should be given and what the alternatives are, an appropriate decision cannot be made and the patient cannot protect his own best interest. He must find another doctor!

2. Examination and Diagnosis

A. History of your complaint

Organize your thoughts before going to the doctor so that you can get the most out of your time with him. He will want to know "When it started," "The nature of the condition, (pain is bad in the morning, comes and goes, is getting progressively worse)," "What you've done about it, both self-care and professionally," and "the results of these treatments." He may also ask if you have any related problems (knee, hip, back, etc.) He will also want to have a medical history that covers any major illnesses, operations, injuries, hospitalizations, or allergies that you may have experienced and any medications that you may be taking. The doctor will appreciate your interest in yourself and will be more interested in you if you take the time in advance to have this information available.

B. Examination

Your doctor will touch or move the painful areas. Cooperate fully with him and answer his questions. He may examine other areas that you feel are unrelated to your problem to aid him in his diagnosis. He also may look at your other (not painful) foot to compare it to the painful one.

C. X-rays

Where foot pain is concerned, the benefits of an x-ray far outweigh the risk. (Although the public concern for unnecessary x-rays is totally justifiable, since one-fourth of the body's bones are in the feet, x-rays are absolutely required for accurate diagnosis). Don't be upset if the doctor also wants an x-ray of the non-painful foot for comparison. What appears to be "abnormal" in one foot may also show up in the other foot and thus be entirely "normal" for you. Accurate foot x-rays should be made with your weight distributed on both feet. If a doctor wants to take an x-ray of your foot while you are seated or on a table . . . ask why!

D. A new diagnostic tool—the EDG *tm*.

The electro-dynagram is a diagnostic computer developed by the Langer Group of Deer Park, New York. Seven sensors, attached to the sole of the feet, measure the pressure put on specific areas of the foot during each phase of the walking step. A sensor is hooked up to a pack that is placed around the patient's waist. The patient walks around for about 30 seconds either with or without shoes. The pack is then plugged into the EDG computer and within minutes a biomechanical printout appears comparing the person's gait to one that is considered "normal."

3. The Plan

Once the examination and diagnosis phase is over, the doctor will come up with a plan of action. It's important to realize that there are many different ways to approach a problem and that the best treatment for one person is not necessarily the best for another. For example, because there are over 100 different operative procedures for bunion correction, where and when your doctor was trained and the nature of his specialty can make a substantial difference in the kind of treatment he will choose. The other critical factor that enters into his decision is you, the patient! Differences in age, temperament, ambition, and fears reflect the fact that no two patients have the same needs. The expectations of a 60 year-old sedentary man cannot be related to those of a 20 year-old marathon runner. You must learn the choices and alternatives from the doctor so that you can make an intelligent decision about what treatment you will receive. A word about second opinions: if your questions are not satisfactorily answered, get a second or third opinion without fail. Keep in mind, however, that it may be very much different than the first doctor's and very confusing. Also be aware that good results can be obtained by many foot doctors using many different methods.

4. The Arsenal

The doctor may treat you conservatively or aggressively, depending on your needs. He may even start out the same way you did when you tried to treat the problem yourself. Therefore, it's important to describe exactly what did and didn't work for you when he takes your history. Fortunately, the doctor also has a few more weapons available for you.

A. Palliation, first-aid

This is temporary relief rendered by a podiatrist to remove the pain from a corn, callous, or ingrown toenail. It is strictly a first-aid treatment and will not get rid of the problem permanently.

B. Mechanical Means

These are the various slings, splints, bandages, crutches, canes, paddings, strappings, and casts that doctors use to "rest" parts of the body that are damaged or over-stressed. Orthotics also fall into this category. These are inserts custom fabricated to each foot for continual wear in all shoes to correct such common problems as limb-length differences and foot imbalances.

C. Physical Therapy

1. Heat and cold used in treating various muscle, tendon, and bone disorders. Heat is generated through the use of a heating pad, diathermy (electrical deep heat) and hydrocollator (moist heat).

2. Electro-therapy

Electrical nerve stimulation—used to stimulate muscle groups damaged by injury, disease, or surgery. Relieves swelling and eases pain.

TENS-Transcutaneous Nerve Stimulation—Similar to the above, TENS uses electrical stimulation to ease pain. It is very portable and easy to use.

Paraffin Bath

Paraffin wax heated to 140 degrees. The part is immersed in the hot wax, removed and dipped several times allowing a coating of deep penetrating heat. Wonderful treatment for arthritis and post-operative care.

Whirlpool Bath

A relaxing modality that speeds up circulation to the extremities. This promotes healing and the removal of tissue waste products from the body.

Ultra Sound

High-frequency sound waves are used to reduce inflammation. It is our personal belief that electrical nerve stimulation and TENS is better for this purpose.

D. Medications

These are the oral and injectable medications of the doctor's arsenal. Make sure you understand any side effects and risks that might occur as well as why the particular drug was chosen for your condition and what benefits you are expected to derive by taking it.

E. Surgery

Surgery is one of the most effective ways to influence the course of foot disorders, but as is the case with most other treatments, it can change the course of a problem for the worse as well as for the better. Moreover, the side effects and complications of surgery are prompt and often irreversible. Because of the dramatic nature of a foot operation, patients quite rightly have innate fears, and these must be allayed. This is why the choice of a doctor is critical. Patients who face corrective treatment of a foot problem have both the right and the responsibility to ask questions. It is your body, and you must make the final decision about surgery. If the level of communication with your doctor is poor, or you do not have the facts you need to make a proper decision, you must either clarify this situation with your doctor or find another doctor.

If you require a surgical operation, the most important thing to remember—no matter what your doctor tells you—is that there is no such thing as minor surgery. Any time an anesthetic is used so that somebody can slice you open and play with things inside of you, making a recovery necessary, you're opening yourself up to a multitude of potential problems. Most people are afraid of surgery but accept it when it's presented to them. The most important thing for the patient to decide is: is the surgery necessary in the first place? Take a good hard look at the surgeon who is going to operate on you before you put yourself in his hands. It is also a good idea to talk to people that he has operated on in the past. A surgeon should have no reservations about allowing you to talk to patients on whom he has performed surgery. If he does, run—quickly. And ask for a second opinion—or a third opinion, if necessary—and study the doctor's reaction to your request. If he "needs" the surgery more than you do, you're both in trouble. Although this may be confusing to you, if you are really in doubt, it's better to delay the surgery until you are positive that it's for you. Remember the final decision on matters affecting your health should always be yours, not the doctor's.

a. Major Foot Surgery

This is foot surgery where both feet are to be done at the same time to correct a multitude of problems. Your best bet for this type of surgery is a foot surgeon with judgment, technical skill, and humane qualities, who operates in a community hospital of several hundred beds, and who is board-certified by the American Board of Podiatric Surgery.

b. Ambulatory Foot Surgery

This type of foot surgery is performed in an office or an outpatient surgical center. Again, we would choose a board-certified foot surgeon for this type of surgery. The patient can walk into the surgeon's office and walk out afterwards and can even return to work the same or next day. Usually only one or two procedures are done on a single foot for best results. If a surgeon wants to do 40 procedures on you in his office, all at the same sitting, on both feet, say goodbye fast.

c. Laser-Beam Surgery

The laser is a device that generates an intense beam of light. This light beam is man-made and is not known to occur in nature. Although laser surgery has only been around for the past 10 or 12 years, new uses are being found for it daily. The laser beam vaporizes diseased tissue without hurting the surrounding tissues. There is no x-ray exposure when using the laser beam. Patients report very little pain after laser beam surgery, and follow-up care is much less than with conventional surgery. Laser surgery can be done in the office, in the hospital, or in an outpatient facility and can only be used for SOFT-TISSUE SURGERY. It cannot yet be used for bone surgery. If someone should tell you they are going to do a bunionectomy or bone procedure with laser surgery, put on your running shoes and run out of the office as quickly as possible. Some of the things that we use laser beam surgery for in podiatry are warts, fungus nails, hypertrophied nails, ingrown toenails, skin tumors, tumors within the foot, neuromas, and other soft-tissue growths. Again, it cannot be used for bone surgery. It can, however, be used to make incisions in the foot in conjunction with conventional instruments for bone surgery.

A wide variety of factors should be weighed when surgery is being considered. 1. Clear communication with your doctor is essential. 2. Once you have had the operation, proper rehabilitation is the key to complete surgical success. 3. As a patient, your cooperation and hard work are essential to ultimate surgical success. 4. Although no surgery is guaranteed, with your cooperation and a well-qualified surgeon, your chances of achieving a good result are excellent.

Appendix F

General Foot Hygiene

1. Keep your feet clean. Wash them daily in warm soap and water. Be especially careful to clean between your toes.
2. Dry them carefully, especially in between the toes. Do not rub with a coarse towel.
3. If the skin appears to be especially dry, apply a moisturizing cream to your feet daily. You can use a vegetable shortening, cocoa butter, vitamin A cream, or a mixture of 50% liquid Crisco and 50% VASELINE.™
4. Apply powder to your feet, especially in between the toes, before you put on your socks.
   A. You can also put some powder in your shoes. Johnson & Johnson medicated powder, talcum powder, or any basic dusting powder will do.
5. Make sure when purchasing shoes that you are properly fitted. See Appendix C—Shoes.
6. Keep your shoes in good repair. If the heels, soles, or uppers get worn too much, have them fixed or replace them.
7. If the shoes get wet, or if your feet perspire a good deal, you should give them 12 to 24 hours to air out and dry out thoroughly.
   a. Spray Desenex spray in them or sprinkle with a typical mild dusting powder before you use them.
8. Wear appropriate shoes for specific activities.
   A. Running shoes for brisk walking, jogging and/or running.
   B. Sneakers for basketball.
   C. Tennis shoes for tennis and racquet sports.
   D. Hiking boots for mountain climbing.
9. Always wear only your own shoes, sneakers, and/or slippers. Athlete's Foot and other foot infections can be transmitted through shoe wear.
   A. Discarded, worn down shoes from the previous wearer can only cause the new wearer problems—See Appendix C—Shoes.

10. Wear properly fitted socks or stockings. Do not use tube socks that are made for multiple sizes.

A. Socks or stockings should be ½-inch to ¾-inch longer than the foot. Your toes should have plenty of room to wiggle around.

B. Change your socks daily.

C. You may have to change socks several times a day, especially if your feet perspire excessively or you have an odor. See chapter 13 "Sweaty and Smelly Feet."

11. Wear shoes on all hard surfaces. City streets and parks can be littered with broken glass, nails, debris that could become embedded in the bottom of the foot. You may also contract skin and fungus infections from walking barefoot on dirty streets.

12. Barefooted walking is safest on soft, sandy beaches, clean grassy areas, thick carpet, etc.

13. Make sure you have the most comfortable shoes you can on-the-job, especially if you spend most of your time on your feet.

A. Certain industrial workers or construction workers are often required to wear safety shoes.

B. If you're not required to wear safety shoes, it is still advisable to get shoes with thick, strong heel-counters and thick cushioned soles if you constantly work on hard surfaces.

C. Excessively high-heeled shoes (heel heighths of 4 inches or more), really shouldn't be worn on the job if you stand most of the time. If you insist, then at least rotate heel heighths. By rotating heel heighths you give the muscles in the back of the leg a chance to stretch a little bit. You also do not put as much stress on the front of the leg, feet, and lower back.

D. At night, you might want to wear a sneaker to continue to stretch the calf muscles out.

E. Try some calf muscle stretching or some wall-pushes to stretch out the backs of the calves.

14. Keep the toenails trimmed by cutting them straight across.

A. Use a toenail scissor, nail clipper, or toenail cutter that has been washed in soap and water and rinsed in a recognized antiseptic.

B. Put 2 tablespoons of mild household detergent into a gallon of warm water. Soak your foot or feet for 10 minutes.

C. Then, carefully cut your nails straight across.

D. Dry thoroughly and apply an antiseptic spray or liquid to any nail or nails that you may have nicked or that drew blood. (This is a good idea to do in any case.) Feel free to do this for all of your nails.

15. If you have any foot or leg problems—consult the appropriate chapter in this book and try to alleviate the condition or conditions by yourself. Follow all the programs closely.

16. If you cannot help yourself, then consult a podiatrist, with new and improved techniques most problems can be permanently relieved.

17. If your feet get cold at night, wear socks, use extra blankets, and raise the thermostat. Do not go to bed with a heating pad or hot water bottle.

18. Do not use medicated corn pads or other remedies commercially available unless recommended in this book for the appropriate condition, or unless recommended by your podiatrist.

Index